The Impact of Genetic
Hearing Impairment

The Impact of Genetic Hearing Impairment

Edited by

DAFYDD STEPHENS FRCP

Cardiff University

and

LESLEY JONES PhD

Hull/York Medical School

University of Leeds

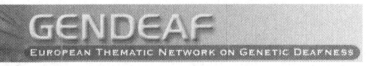

GENDEAF

EUROPEAN THEMATIC NETWORK ON GENETIC DEAFNESS

W

WHURR PUBLISHERS

LONDON AND PHILADELPHIA

© 2005 Whurr Publishers Ltd

First published 2005 by Whurr Publishers Ltd
19b Compton Terrace, London N1 2UN, England and
325 Chestnut Street, Philadelphia PA 19106, USA

British Library Cataloguing in Publication Data

A catalogue record for this book is available from the
British Library.

ISBN 1 86156 437 6

Contents

Contributors

Berth Danermark is Professor of Sociology, Örebro University, Sweden. He is head of the postgraduate school at the Swedish Institute of Disability Research. His main research focus is on communication disorders. He has published books and articles on sociological and psychosocial aspects of hearing impairment. In his research, he has also focused on the rehabilitation process for people with hearing impairment.
e-mail: berth.danermark@ivo.oru.se

Jill Jones was educated in her local mainstream school. She qualified as a Social Worker with Deaf People and has worked in social work settings in local authorities and the NDCS, as well as teaching literacy and Deaf-related subjects. She took a Disability Living Allowance appeal case to the House of Lords, which subsequently became a watershed case in terms of deaf adults and young people being able to make successful claims. She was co-founder and then the Chair of the Deaf Ex-Mainstreamers' Group (DEX), which is an organization campaigning for sign bilingual education in mainstream schools. She now works as the Project Manager for DEX. e-mail: jilljones@dex.org.uk

Lesley Jones is Senior Lecturer in Social Policy and Social Work at Hull/York Medical School and Senior Research Fellow at the Centre for Research in Primary Care, School of Medicine, University of Leeds. She has published widely in the area of people's experience of deafness and of health services, as well as in deaf studies and ethnicity.
e-mail: lesleyg@onetel.net.uk

Sophia Kramer is a psychologist, who has been working at the Department of Audiology at the Vrije University Medical Centre in Amsterdam since 1993. Her major research interests are in psychosocial effects of hearing impairment in adults and methods of assessment. Further interests are in the development of training programmes in audiological rehabilitation. She is involved in various national and international research projects and has published papers on psychosocial aspects of hearing loss, self-report outcome measures and other methods of assessment. She is a fellow of the International Collegium of Rehabilitative Audiology (ICRA). e-mail: SE.Kramer@vumc.nl

Patricia Lago-Avery is a National Certified Counsellor whose career in deaf education spans 27 years, 23 years being at the National Technical Institute for the Deaf/Rochester Institute of Technology (NTID/RIT), where she worked as a counsellor and professor. The last 13 years at NTID she specialized in working with students who had secondary disabilities, many of which were visual impairments. Since leaving NTID/RIT she has worked to improve the quality of life of adults and children who are deafblind, at local, national and international levels. Patti chairs the Deaf Blind Collaborative Committee in Rochester, New York as well as serving on the Helen Keller National Center Consumer Advisory Board. e-mail: pllnbu@ritvax.edu

Nele Lemkens is a medical practitioner who is currently completing her training as an ENT specialist. Since 2001 she has been investigating the influence of genetic and environmental factors on age-related hearing impairment and otosclerosis as a part of her PhD programme. The research was performed in the ENT department and the Department of Medical Genetics of Antwerp University. Her main focus is the audiological and clinical picture of age-related hearing impairment and otosclerosis. She has published papers on the audiology and the epidemiology of age-related hearing impairment. e-mail: Nele.Lemkens@pandora.be

Anna Middleton is a Registered Genetic Counsellor working at Addenbrooke's Hospital, Cambridge. Her research has focused on the attitudes of deaf people and their families towards the impact of deafness on the family and attitudes towards prenatal testing for deafness. She is particularly interested in the views of culturally Deaf people towards genetics and the process of genetic counselling for deafness. Anna has written papers and book chapters on her research within the clinical genetics and genetic counselling literature. e-mail: anna.middleton@addenbrookes.nhs.uk

Kerstin Möller is a doctoral candidate at the Swedish Institute of Disability Research, Örebro University, Sweden. She has a master's degree in the Management of Health and Welfare Organizations. Her research focus is on deafblindness. She has conducted public investigations of services for people with deafblindness on behalf of the Swedish Ministry of Social Affairs as well as the the Swedish National Agency for Education. She has also worked as a research assistant in a project developing technical aids for people with deafblindness. e-mail: kerstin.moller@ ivo.oru.se

Wanda Neary is a Consultant Community Paediatrician (Audiology) working in Warrington, England. She has collaborated closely with the Manchester NF2 Team since 1989 and has published papers jointly on the clinical and genetic aspects of NF2. She has a particular interest in the audiological aspects of NF2. She is currently carrying out a research study into the quality of life in NF2. e-mail: wandaneary@hotmail.com

Dafydd Stephens is an audiological physician and Professor of Audiological Medicine in Cardiff University. His main clinical and research interest is in audiological rehabilitation. His interest in genetics dates back to his schooldays and has been furthered recently by his active involvement in three European Union projects in the field. He has published widely in these areas and on the history of medicine. e-mail: stephensd@cf.ac.uk

Additional and significant contributions were received from:

Michael Baser is a geneticist and neurofibromatosis 2 expert, Los Angeles.

Gareth Evans is a clinical geneticist and co-leader of the Manchester neuro-fibromatosis 2 progamme.

Richard Ramsden is a pioneer in auditory brainstem implants and co-leader of the Manchester neurofibromatosis 2 programme.

Preface

This book sets out to examine the social and psychological effects of genetic deafness, hearing impairment and the genetic interventions associated with them. There have been enormous developments in this area over the last 20 years, and the book reflects some of those changes in the lives of deaf people and those who live and work with them. Scientific progress in the study of genetic deafness has meant that ethical, political and economic dilemmas have entered the field of what was once seen as an area of objective, value-free endeavour. These issues cannot be avoided and we seek to address them in a straightforward way by making use of different perspectives within the book; medical, psychological and sociological as well as personal and political.

The book arises from the European Union GENDEAF Thematic Network project, and is a product of the Psychosocial Working Group of that project, which attempts to bridge the gap between the service users' organizations and those concerned with clinical and molecular genetics.

Although the study and practice of medical genetics and of the genetics of hearing impairment might be seen as essentially socially neutral topics of scientific endeavour, the actual effects have by no means been neutral. This applies particularly to the way in which the findings are used and applied by clinicians, teachers, politicians and other professionals involved with people with hearing impairments.

Such misuse of the scientific findings relating to genetic hearing impairment goes back a long way, and one of its greatest perpetrators was a key figure in the field of education of the Deaf, Alexander Graham Bell. Despite having a deaf wife, he very much espoused the eugenic concepts of Galton, aimed at eliminating such 'defects' from the population. This was carried to extremes under National Socialism in Germany in the 1930s with initially sterilization and later 'elimination' of individuals with congenital deafness.

It is not surprising, therefore, that many Deaf people are suspicious of developments in the study of genetic hearing impairment which, via prenatal diagnosis and subsequent termination of pregnancy or by gene therapy, they

xii — The Impact of Genetic Hearing Impairment

feel could lead to the elimination of people with congenital deafness. This is reinforced by the statements of some clinicians within genetics, otology and audiology, categorically proposing the elimination of genetic deafness.

The concepts held both by Deaf people and by some professionals are false in that only some 50% of congenital hearing impairment is genetically determined. Furthermore, over 36 different genes, mutations of which can result in non-syndromal hearing impairment, have so far been identified, and many more have been localized. Approximately half of these are generally associated with recessive inheritance. In addition, the entrenched views of some professions ignores the social impact of human rights' legislation, the growth of the political disability movement, and the increasing recognition and status of the Deaf community and of national sign languages. In this book, we try to maintain a balance between the medical and social models of disability by not focusing on the impairment as 'the problem' but taking into account the impact of the barriers to communication and access created by others. Obviously each author has their own perspective and the readers must make up their own minds. We simply present informed views within the rapidly changing field of genetic interventions in hearing impairment in the hope of providing some insight into improving policy and practice in an important area.

Our research in this area has also highlighted the dearth of knowledge and understanding about the impact on individuals and their families of having genetic or familial hearing impairment. As previously mentioned, only a very small proportion of genetic hearing impairment is congenital, accounting for some 50% of congenital hearing impairment. This amounts to less than 1 per 1000 of the population. However, some 15–20% of the population have a significant hearing impairment, mainly of late onset, and recent twin studies indicate that approximately 50% of that is also genetically determined. Furthermore, although we know a little about the impact of having a family history of hearing impairment in children, there is a complete dearth of knowledge of such an impact in adults. This book was originally intended to be an overview of the psychosocial effects of genetic hearing impairment in particular, as opposed to hearing impairment in general. However, because of the absence of information specifically on that topic, the four key chapters on the impact of genetic hearing impairment in children, working-age adults, elderly people and the deafblind have had to concentrate on the impact of such conditions in general, while highlighting any specific evidence of the impact of genetic conditions.

In addition to these four key areas, we have also included a consideration of otosclerosis, one of the few genetic causes of hearing impairment which is amenable to surgical treatment, and of neurofibromatosis 2 (NF2), a condition that causes hearing impairment but is also potentially lethal.

Finally, we include two autobiographical chapters outlining the experiences and impact on the lives of the authors of having a genetic hearing impairment and genetic deafblindness.

The book begins with two chapters on responses to genetic deafness and the growth of genetic intervention. The first, by Lesley Jones, a social scientist who has worked for many years in the field of Deaf studies, examines the social aspects of genetics and deafness and particularly the response of the Deaf community. Anna Middleton, a genetic counsellor, reviews her own and other studies on the attitudes of Deaf and hearing parents towards genetic interventions, including new data from her own studies.

We then move on to two methodological chapters providing the structure for the overviews on the impact of the hearing impairment and related conditions covered in the main part of the book. In the first of these Dafydd Stephens, an audiological physician, and Berth Danermark, a sociologist, present the relevant parts of the World Health Organization's International Classification of Functioning, Disability and Health (ICF) which we have adopted as the framework for examining the impact of genetic hearing impairment. This model attempts to bridge the medical and social models of disability, so seems particularly appropriate to our approach. The next chapter, by Berth Danermark, Sophia Kramer (a psychologist) and Dafydd Stephens, outlines the general methodological approach adopted in the three review chapters on the impact of hearing impairment in general, and of genetic hearing impairment in particular.

In the first of these review chapters, Dafydd Stephens examines the impact of hearing impairment on children, particularly those with moderate-to-profound congenital disorders, who have been the most extensively studied. There is also, however, increasing evidence of a significant impact of mild and unilateral hearing impairments. While there is little information on the impact of genetic deafness *per se*, there is a body of literature indicating that the children of deaf parents, probably mainly with autosomal dominant inheritance, experience the impairment differently, with less impact on their self-esteem than the deaf children of hearing parents.

Berth Danermark then provides an extensive overview of the effect of hearing impairment on adults of working age, hitherto a very neglected area, and is able to identify only very limited information on the impact of a family history in this respect.

Similarly, Sophia Kramer, drawing together the very diverse results on the effects of hearing impairment in elderly people, is unable to identify any studies on the impact of such a family history. She does, however, highlight many methodological weaknesses of existing studies, emphasizing the need for a more systematic approach.

Kerstin Möller, a health services researcher, reviews the situation with regard to deafblindness, an area bedevilled with definitional problems. These stem, in part, from the variability of both the hearing and the visual impairments, their age of onset and their progression. This applies, in particular, to Usher syndrome, a genetic condition of sensorineural hearing impairment and retinitis pigmentosa, which recent genetic studies have shown covers a range of mutations in different genes, with very variable phenotypes. However, despite this she has admirably drawn the literature together and highlighted the deficits in our knowledge.

Nele Lemkens, an academic otologist, looks at the impact of otosclerosis, and finds that patients' expectations are very much conditioned by the possibility of surgery for the condition. However, although the condition is common, there has been little work on its impact, probably because most surgeons have little interest beyond the functional results of their intervention.

Wanda Neary, a paediatric audiological physician, addresses the effects of NF2. This has multisystem effects, resulting from tumours in different parts of the central nervous system, including those affecting both cochlear nerves. Surprisingly the psychosocial impact of the condition has been almost completely neglected and the chapter has had to concentrate on the background of the condition and the impact of related disorders.

Finally, we have two important autobiographical studies by individuals with hearing impairment who have themselves become professionally involved in the field. The first, by Patricia Lago-Avery, a counsellor, deals with the development of different components of Usher syndrome and her experience of having a cochlear implant. The second, by Jill Jones, a social worker and researcher, gives a personal perspective on genetic deafness caused by Treacher Collins syndrome. These two accounts provide valuable insights that could inform and improve practice.

The book concludes with a glossary, which all authors have attempted to adhere to throughout their overviews, deviating only when quoting the work of others.

We hope this overview will be useful in stimulating more focused work in this field. Already, most of the authors have been conducting specific studies to fill some of the gaps, but much more needs to be done by all interested researchers and clinicians. We are convinced of the value of multidisciplinary work in this area in order to address the issues raised by the rapid changes taking place in the experience, theory and practice of genetic hearing impairment. Research in the field cannot be done in isolation from the very real psychosocial effects on the daily lives of people with genetic hearing impairments if it is to adequately inform the policy and practice of the relevant professionals. We hope that this book goes some way towards doing that by drawing together some important elements of the relevant work.

Dafydd Stephens
Lesley Jones
October 2004

Acknowledgement

This book is published with the support of the European Commission, Fifth Framework programme, Quality of Life and Management of Living resources programme. The authors and editors are solely responsible for this publication. It does not represent the opinion of the Community. The Community is not responsible for any use that might be made of the data appearing therein.

CHAPTER 1
Future perfect: social aspects of genetics and deafness

LESLEY JONES

When a Deaf lesbian couple in the United States used a sperm donor, a deaf friend with five generations of deafness in his family, in order to create a deaf child of their own, the *BMJ* described it as 'designer disability' (Savulescu, 2002). This is one area where the science of genetics and the personal politics of deafness collide.

Ladd, a deaf researcher, (2003) described the discovery of the deaf gene as being 'the final solution', echoing National Socialism in 1930s' Germany. For many Deaf people, genetics is seen as just that, as a way of 'getting rid' of deaf people. In order to look closely at deafness and genetics, we have to set it in the context of genetics generally. It is a discipline with a troubled history and one that needs careful consideration. In this chapter we will consider the biomedical and social aspects of genetics, new and old, and also the impact of genetic medicine on deaf people's lives in particular, and the social issues raised by genetics and their implications for people working in medicine in the field of audiology.

Genetics

Genetics may not be the wonder science that the media make it out to be, and, like any other technology, genetic engineering has its pluses and its minuses. The discovery that a gene can be isolated and its function identified and then reproduced does not mean that all our health problems are solved. The title of this chapter, 'Future perfect', refers to the idea of DNA as the 'book of life' or the 'grammar of life', as it is often referred to in the literature. The reality of genetics though, as opposed to the myth, is likely to be more complex than the offer of perfection portrayed in the Star Wars film *The Attack of the Clones*.

If genetics can be seen as accounting for the differences between people and how we explain them in biomedical terms, we can look at these claims and the offer of opportunities in order to control them. These differences might be about height, skin colour, temperament, disease – a wide spectrum. For example, some scientists have referred to the 'gay gene', the 'alcoholic gene', even the 'love of the sea' gene (as in the nineteenth-century term *thalassophilia*, used as an explanation for sea captains' love of the sea). Deafness fits into this context by being a difference which has social as well as biomedical implications.

A gene can be seen quite straightforwardly as a unit of inheritance, but another view is that genetic determinism will decide our future, when we might die and what we might die of. The possibility of prediction generates uncertainties and anxieties, so, as a social scientist and not a geneticist, I want to look at the relationship between the biomedical and social aspects of genetics and deafness. Is it an 'either or' or is it a 'both and' as Shakespeare and Kerr (2003) describe it?

The interface between genetics and social science

The biomedical explanatory system of genetics is rooted in biology and the natural sciences, whereas the social model is based on social interactions: for example, a person's IQ can be regarded as being explained by inheritance, but others might see it as being explained by education and opportunity, as in the nature and nurture arguments about child development.

Social science is sometimes seen as opinion and speculation, but is biomedical science value-free? Is it objective existing in a vacuum, separate from society? Ann Oakley (1993), for example, looked at the birth weights of babies and found that not even this could be seen as objectively removed from human error or by the differences in the way in which people measured. The size of women's brains and of people from different ethnic groups has been given as biomedical explanation of difference, relying solely on biology illustrating the complex relationship between 'fact' and 'predjudices'.

Dreptomania, a slave's desire to run away from their master, was classified as a disease in the USA in the nineteenth century. Physicians actually believed that it was a medical condition. This reflected the views of the dominant group in the USA at the time, just as homosexuality was still seen as a pathological disease up until the 1960s, also reflecting a view of a dominant minority.

So is science, and genetics in particular, value-free? It is useful to consider who has a stake in genetics. Scientists, clinicians, bioethicists, social scientists, patient interest groups and industry all have a stake in it at present. Deaf people in particular are a good example of an interest group in this context.

One natural scientist sees it in the following way: 'Genetics is now the "big science" and an alliance between venture capital and academia' (Rose,

2001). The questions to ask are, does genetics offer a reduction in disease, increased life expectancy and an end to global poverty and famine? Does it offer perfect health or only commercial profit? This relationship between 'big science' and academia affects cochlear implants and neonatal screening for deafness, as well as the manufacture of hearing aids and environmental aids and in addition to genetic engineering.

'Old' and 'new' genetics

Generally 'old genetics' refers to a period before 1973 (and work in genetics and deafness comes largely after that period). Historically there are, however, contextual aspects of deafness that are important in genetics.

The ability to make copies of DNA sequences was an important step. The growth of the Human Genome Project and genetic screening, gene therapy, cloning and genetically modified crops are also seen as part of the new genetics. A genome is all the genetic material in the chromosomes of an organism (23 pairs of chromosomes in the human genome). The Human Genome Project, a multinational project, began in the USA in the 1980s to collect and analyse human genetic material. In 1998, the Icelandic database (and Biobank UK in 2003) created controversy over a public/private venture to collect these human genetic records and material, originally to study disease. Iceland was chosen as a relatively small, isolated and homogeneous community. Arguments about infringement of individual freedom and 'selling the family secrets' have made this a controversial area.

The new genetics is sometimes seen as 'inheritance strikes back' after the troubled history of the old genetics. Mendel's nineteenth-century work on dominant and recessive genes in plants and the work of Darwin's cousin, Galton, on inherited genius gave rise to eugenics. The history of the Eugenics Movement is very firmly linked to the history of deafness. The Eugenics Movement gave genetics a bad name because of its connection with genocide and the selective breeding of workers for the industrial society. Western industrial society in the nineteenth century needed fit workers. After the Boer War soldiers were also needed, and the Infant Welfare Act of 1911, seen as for 'the good of the people', was also to ensure that the poor were fit to fight as well as to work. In nineteenth-century Britain, workers and non-workers were categorized as the poor, the feeble-minded and the criminals, who are now sometimes described as 'the sad, the mad and the bad'. Deaf people were very firmly categorized with the feeble-minded and were seen as unfit for work, although in fact many of them did work.

In the 1920s the Eugenics Movement extended these ideals into who was allowed to reproduce, based on selective breeding. The issue that emerged as important was who decided who was allowed to reproduce. Target groups such as the upper middle classes were seen as being suitable for reproduction as opposed to the unsuitable – the poor or those with some impairment.

In the USA, the Immigration Act (1924) was overtly intended to prevent disease coming into the country. Its effect was to restrict immigration from southern Europe, because people from that region were seen as bringing disease. There are similarities with the views expressed of the asylum seekers and refugees coming into western Europe now, bringing diseases such as TB into these countries.

National Socialism in Germany in the 1930s took genetic purification a further step towards producing a pure Aryan race, excluding not only Jewish people, but gay and lesbian people, gypsies, those with impairments and deaf people in particular. Deaf people were sterilized within schools for deaf children, but they were also taken to concentration camps and 'eliminated'. Getting rid of unwanted characteristics was seen as purifying the race, and this has given the Eugenics Movement, and therefore genetics, a bad name.

The Eugenics Movement is firmly identified in the minds of deaf people as being a part of their oppression by hearing people. Paddy Ladd cites the wearing of blue ribbons. These were worn by deaf people during the war, very much in the way that pink stars were worn by homosexual people, and yellow stars by Jewish people. Throughout his book (2003), Ladd constantly refers back to National Socialism in Germany.

The impact of the old genetics on deafness and Deaf history is clear. It is firmly identified in the minds of Deaf people as being a part of genetic cleansing (Mannion, 1997) and allied with that history. The blue ribbon ceremony at the World Federation of the Deaf in 2002 was entirely based on this resonance with the threat of National Socialism.

The impact of the new genetics

So that is the impact of old genetics. What about the impact of the new genetics on deaf people? From 1989, it became possible to identify a single gene and identify its function. These developments led to genetic testing and screening, and to gene therapy, slower but pharmaceutically more rapid. The problem is how the new genetics affects people's lives and, in particular, deaf people's lives. Genetic testing and screening have particular relevance to deaf people at present: gene therapy is still some way off in this field.

The identification of a gene in isolation, for example the cystic fibrosis gene, is unusual. Only 5% of disease is based on a single gene. Most diseases are polygenic, caused by a number of genes or by a complex interaction between genes and the environment. 'Heredity pulls the gun and the environment pulls the trigger', as one US health promotion programme in the Human Genome Project states. Sometimes there is a multifactorial cause within the womb, sometimes it is the influence of life. The Human Genome Project stresses environmental factors, such as sunlight, tobacco and alcohol, which are part of a very complex picture. The message which the gene sends to the cells is garbled by these different influences. Given that the world is full of these stresses, genetics may only be one of a number of factors in disease.

This multifactorial nature of genetic influence on disease is particularly relevant for deaf people from minority ethnic communities, where consanguinity, for example, is sometimes isolated as a factor influencing the birth of deaf children more than any other. Without any clear access to information about the complex genetic picture, many south Asian people (Chamba et al., 1988) feel that white health professionals place too much emphasis on consanguinity, and that the complex nature of deafness and genetics has never really been explained to them.

Limitations of genetics

Doubts about the universal panacea notion of genetics are raised among geneticists as well as other groups. Strohman, a microbiologist, summarizes these doubts:

> We have wrongly extended the theory of the gene to another area altogether. We have been lulled into reasoning that if the gene theory works at one level, from DNA to protein, it must work at all higher levels as well. We have thus extended the theory of the gene to the role of gene management, but gene management is an entirely different process involving interactive cellular processes that display a complexity that may be described only as trans-calculational, a mathematical term for 'mind-boggling' (2000, p. 104).

He goes on to say

> Whilst the simple storybook explanations provide a model of something akin to a gene machine, it is argued that the cell is beginning to look more like a complex, adaptive system rather than a factory floor of robotic gene machines (p. 108).

So doubts about genetics are expressed from within the scientific and genetic community, as well as by interest groups and social scientists. Others disagree, of course. For example, Dawkins (1976) argued for the gene machine absolutely.

The impact of genetics on deaf people

So what is the impact of genetics on the lives of deaf people and those who work with them? Screening has a huge impact in the selection and elimination of characteristics such as deafness. The two types of screening, to identify carriers before conception and fetal characteristics after conception, have changed lives. Screening before conception – for sickle cell anaemia, for example – does not exist independently. It exists alongside a complicated picture, particularly for sickle cell anaemia, of racism, lack of understanding and lack of access to information. The second type, screening for fetal characteristics after conception, for example for Down's syndrome or muscular dystrophy, affects people's lives because testing means that risk surveillance increases. Does it help for example to tell a 19-year-old that they might get Alzheimer's when they are 75 while they might be run over by a bus when they are 20?

The knowledge of a tendency to the late-onset diseases such as Alzheimer's or Huntington's disease, or breast or colon cancer, means that identify is altered throughout life. There are examples of women having elective mastectomies because there is breast cancer in the family. Discrimination often results in difficulties with insurance arrangements and with employers. Hidden or latent disabilities have even more of an impact. This knowledge can be seen as 'toxic knowledge'.

Risk surveillance testing is often justified in two ways: cost-effectiveness and informed choice. The social implication of testing carries with it an idea that all disabled people are a drain on society (Shakespeare and Kerr, 2003). Yet, if we look at examples such as President Roosevelt of the USA, Stephen Hawking and David Blunkett (admittedly all white, high-status men), they are examples of people who have an impairment and who have yet contributed to life, so this simply is not true.

David Colley, a disabled activist (cited in Shakespeare, 2003), writes:

> Disabled people have everything to fear from the new genetics. At worst it is our very existence; we will be eliminated simply as 'genetic spelling mistakes' once again referring to the 'book of life' and 'grammar of life' notion of genetics.

At best we will be reinforced as biological abnormalities, as defective human beings.

Testing will not eliminate disability. Only 1% of disability is from birth, and one in eight of the population is disabled; a lot of disability happens later on in life. Shakespeare and Kerr (2003) write 'You could see it in a more positive light, that previous statistic that we are all disabled now'.

The association of the Human Genome Project with the idea of the perfect human genome is a platonic fallacy. DNA copying is fallible; the 'spelling mistakes' will always be there. We all have limitations at birth, which could cause disease from the minute we are born. We all carry alleles for four or five recessive conditions within our genomes which could cause cystic fibrosis or sickle cell anaemia in our children. The DNA in each cell is also bombarded with things that might cause it to mutate and its repair mechanisms decrease so that, as we grow older, one in four people may develop cancer (Kirkwood, 2000). Genetics not only makes it clear that this perfection is a myth, it also emphasizes our own frailty and our lack of immortality, and our imperfections and inequalities are highlighted.

There is another problem implicit in genetic counselling: ensuring that all the information offered to patients is accurate and relevant. Is the genetic counselling that people receive about deafness always based on the best information? Are value judgements being made? Is there an assumption that some people are more suitable to reproduce? That is exactly why the Deaf lesbian couple's choice to have a deaf child throws a different light on the matter. Deaf parents very often are delighted to have a deaf child, and disappointed to have a hearing child (Ladd, 2003). This is well known, and something that needs careful thought.

'Free market eugenics' has given rise to the idea of genetic engineering and of designer babies, designer disability and the ability to choose by ability to pay for choice. The lesbian couple previously mentioned is an example of this. Are we engineering perfection? Are babies going to be selected by the colour of their eyes, the colour of their hair, their gender, their intelligence, their physical perfection? Do designer babies mean that having that kind of choice is available only to people with money?

Gene piracy is another issue.

> If the Vampire Project goes ahead and patents are put on genetic material from Aboriginal people, this would be legalised theft. Over the last 200 years, non-Aboriginal people have taken our land, our language, culture and health – even our children. Now they want to take the genetic material which makes us Aboriginal people as well (Nason, 1994).

Aboriginal people see this as legalized theft, and it has some similarities with how deaf people see cochlear implants and genetic testing as being genocide for them by getting rid of deaf people.

Biocolonialism and ownership of genes have implications for deaf people and for medicine. What is perfection? Who decides what we die of eventually? Who has access to genetic technologies and who makes these choices? Is this dystopic bio-fantasy the future?

> By 2350 The GenRich, who account for ten percent of the American population, all carry synthetic genes, genes that were created in the laboratory. The GenRich are a modern-day hereditary class of genetic aristocrats, all aspects of the economy, the media, the entertainment industry and the knowledge industry are controlled by members of the GenRich class, Naturals work as low-paid service providers or as labourers (Silver, 1998).

As time passes:

> The GenRich class and the Natural class will become the GenRich humans and the Natural humans – entirely separate species with no ability to cross-breed and with as much romantic interest in each other as a current human would have for a chimpanzee.

In the film *Galactica* (2000), there is a genetic underclass of people who are not pure genetically and are discriminated against.

Implications

So what are the implications for the future for deaf people?

* Will individuals be identified as predisposed to a particular disease?
* Will new drugs be devised to alter genes?
* Will immunotherapy techniques develop further?
* Will there be avoidance of environmental conditions?
* Will there be replacement of defective genes, through gene therapy?
* Will there be a move from treatment of the sick to prevention of disease?
* Does deafness count as a disease?

The last is the major point that we have to address here, for people who have grown up deaf, people who identify themselves as part of the Deaf community, part of Deaf Culture or the Deaf Nation. Deafness is not seen as a disease by many deaf people: they see themselves as a linguistic minority, living valuable, useful lives, contributing to society. Is there any reason that they should ever see themselves as something that needs to be eliminated, to be got rid of?

The deaf world's relationship with genetics will always be a troubled one. Genetics will always be seen, as Ladd (2003) describes it, as 'medical neocolonialism, experimentation for profit'. It will always be seen as a way of eradicating deaf people. Ladd concludes his book by saying:

> These developments have threatened to turn lay people's attention away from accepting deaf people in communities and back towards curing them.

The complex interaction between the technological and social aspects of genetics in relation to deafness are well illustrated by Blume (1999):

> Thus there are two very different accounts of cochlear implantation, for example, embedded in two very different histories. One is a tale of medicine's triumph, akin to many other such tales: a tale of courageous pioneers, of the wonders of medical science and technology. The other is a genre which has emerged only in the past two decades and which highlights the subordination of medicine to surveillance, social control and normalisation. This tale is of one of the oppression of Deaf people and of hearing people's inability to accept deaf people as they are.

The ambivalence between medicine and deaf people is also illustrated in the relationship between those deaf from birth and those who become deaf, and how different deaf people identify themselves within that relationship

(Jones and Bunton, 2004). These complexities are being played out in the contexts not just of genetic testing and counselling but also of speech therapy, audiology, cochlear implants and surgery.

Conclusions

Medicine and science may offer the notion of restored order, cure, and repair and correction but the reality for deaf people may be more complicated than that. Again, Blume (1999) summarizes this:

> Deaf people have located cochlear implants within a history of their own oppression, rather than in a history of their own progress. Each historical rendering is used to try to influence policy. The contest, however, is an unequal one.

This is referring to cochlear implants, but it applies just as well to genetics.

If we believe the promise of some of the claims of genetics, if not fantasy, there are two visions of the way we will go in the future. One is the future perfect, another is a future imperfect, with an exaggeration of our worst qualities.

References

Blume S (1999) Histories of cochlear implantation. Social Science and Medicine 49: 1257–1268.

Chamba R, Ahmad W, Jones L (1988) Improving Services for Asian Deaf Children: parents and professional's perspectives. Policy Press, Bristol.

Dawkins R (1976) The Selfish Gene. Oxford University Press, Oxford.

Jones L, Bunton R (2004) Wounded or warrior? Stories of being or becoming Deaf. In: Hurwitz B (ed.) Narrative Research in Health and Illness. BMJ Books, London.

Kirkwood TBL (2000) New science for an old problem. Trends in Genetics 18: 441–442.

Ladd P (2003) Understanding Deaf Culture: in search of deafhood. Multilingual Matters, Clevedon.

Mannion M (1997) Genetic cleansing. Journal of the Irish Deaf Society 11(41): 12–13.

Nason D (1994) Tickner warns over Aboriginal gene sampling. The Australian (25 January): 3.

Oakley A (1993) Essays on Women, Medicine and Health. Edinburgh University Press, Edinburgh.

Rose H (2001) The Commodification of Bioinformation: The Icelandic Health Sector Database. Wellcome Trust, London.

Savulescu J (2002) Deaf lesbians, designer disability and the future of medicine. BMJ 324: 771–773.

Shakespeare T (2003) Rights, risks and responsibilities: new genetics and disabled people. In: Birke S, Williams L, Bendelow G (eds) Debating Biology. Routledge, London.

Shakespeare T, Kerr A (2003) Genetic Politics: from eugenics to genome. New Clarion Press, Cheltenham.

Silver LM (1998) Remaking Eden: cloning and beyond in a brave new world. Weidenfeld & Nicolson, London.

Strohman R (2000) Genetic determinism as a failing paradigm in biology and medicine: implications for health and wellness. In: Schneider Jamner M, Stokols D (eds) Promoting Human Wellness: new frontiers for research, practice and policy. University of California Press, Berkeley, CA, pp. 104, 108.

Chapter 2
Parents' attitudes towards genetic testing and the impact of deafness in the family

Anna Middleton

This chapter focuses on the attitudes of parents of deaf children towards genetic testing for deafness and also documents the varied experiences that parents of deaf children have. For example, with regard to how successful the communication is between child and parent, the impact of the deafness on the child, the 'burden of disease', support received, wish for a cure and experience of obtaining a diagnosis and education for the child.

As genetic testing in pregnancy or prenatal genetic diagnosis (PND) for non-life-threatening genetic conditions becomes increasingly possible, it is important to know whether there is potential interest in using such testing. This chapter therefore also aims to gain an understanding of where PND for deafness fits into the scheme of conditions for which prenatal testing is possible, by comparing attitudes towards PND for different conditions.

The following sections look at genetic causes of deafness, the connexin 26 gene, the types of genetic testing for deafness, what genetic counselling is and some of the literature on the impact of deafness on the individual, family and community. Details of a large study of parents' attitudes are also given, the results are presented and a discussion of these follows.

Deafness and genetics

There are many different causes of deafness, including environmental and genetic factors (Cohen and Gorlin, 1995). Of the 1 in 1000–2000 children with severe–profound, congenital or early-onset deafness, approximately 20–60% are thought to be deaf due to genetic causes, 20–40% due to environmental causes and the remainder of unknown cause (Fraser, 1964; Parving, 1984; Newton, 1985).

11

Deafness resulting from **genetic** factors is usually hereditary. Between 59 and 85% cases of genetic deafness are thought to be caused by autosomal recessive genes, 15–33% by autosomal dominant genes and up to 5% by X-linked or mitochondrial genes (Chung and Brown, 1970; Fraser, 1976; Marazita et al., 1993). **Environmental** factors are non-hereditary and include noise damage, rubella or meningitis infection, prematurity and starvation of oxygen at birth. Deafness can also result from the interaction between genes and the environment, such as with aminoglycoside-induced deafness (Prezant et al., 1993).

The connexin 26 gene

Gene faults, 'alterations or mutations' in the *GJB2* or connexin 26 (Cx26) gene are very common, accounting for up to 50% of genetic childhood deafness, with a carrier frequency of 1 in 31 in certain populations (Denoyelle et al., 1997; Estivill et al., 1998; Kelley et al., 1998). One in 10 individuals with sporadic non-syndromal deafness (deafness isolated in the family) has their deafness because of alterations in the Cx26 gene (Lench et al., 1998). Deafness as a result of alterations in Cx26 varies from mild through to profound (Denoyelle et al., 1999).

Genetic testing

Several hundred genes are known to be involved with deafness. It is possible to test for many of these. 'Genetic testing' is a general term that can refer to different types of testing, e.g. diagnostic, carrier, prenatal and predictive.

- **Diagnostic testing** is used to diagnose whether a deaf person has a gene alteration or alterations that are likely to be the cause of their deafness.
- **Carrier genetic testing** tells a hearing individual whether they carry a gene alteration, which, when also carried by their partner, would usually give them, as a couple, a 1 in 4 chance that their child will be deaf.
- **Prenatal genetic testing** tells a pregnant mother via an invasive test, such as amniocentesis or chorionic villus sampling, whether the fetus has a gene alteration(s) that could cause deafness. The invasive test involves an approximately 0.5–1% risk of miscarriage of the pregnancy. Information from a prenatal genetic test could then be used by the parents to decide whether the pregnancy should be continued or not. If not, the mother could have a termination of pregnancy (TOP). Prenatal genetic testing is a form of diagnostic testing but it is performed in the prenatal phase; it is also known as prenatal genetic diagnosis (PND).
- **Predictive genetic testing** could tell a hearing person whether they have a gene alteration that could predispose them to developing deafness later in life.

As more genes linked to deafness are discovered and the research into the molecular genetics of deafness advances, it becomes easier to incorporate genetic testing for deafness within clinical genetics services. Many researchers within the field of molecular genetics are excited by the prospect of rapid incorporation of deafness research into routine clinical practice (Reardon, 1998). However, this should be treated with some caution, since the availability of some services such as PND for deafness elicits much ethical debate about whether deafness is a 'serious' enough condition for PND and whether TOP is an acceptable option for parents who do not want a child of a particular hearing status.

It is becoming increasingly possible to offer genetic testing for non-life-threatening genetic conditions such as deafness. Patients will therefore be faced with more choices relating to PND than ever before. This raises issues about which technologies should be available to families seen for genetic counselling.

Genetic counselling

Genetic counselling can be defined as:

> the process by which patients or relatives at risk of a disorder that may be hereditary are [informed] of the consequences of the disorder, [and] the probability of developing or transmitting it (Harper, 1993)

In addition to the giving of genetic information and the offer of services such as genetic testing, genetic counselling provides emotional support, understanding, listening and help with patients in very personal and sometimes distressing situations. Some people come for genetic counselling with the aim of preventing genetic disorders from being passed on in their family, others come simply for information so that they are better informed of the chances of developing a condition themselves as well as passing one on to their children. Ultimately, any decision, for example, relating to whether to have PND or not is made by the patient; the genetic counsellor's role is to make sure that the patient has all the information available so they can make a decision that is right for them. One of the guiding principles of genetic counselling is 'non-directiveness' (Kessler, 1995); i.e. the geneticist or genetic counsellor does not tell the patient what to do, nor give advice on the decisions they should make. The concept of how appropriate non-directiveness is and whether it is even possible in some situations is frequently discussed within the profession.

With regards to PND for deafness this is not something that is routinely requested within most clinical genetics services in the UK. Therefore it is not a scenario that is well versed among genetic counsellors and geneticists in practice. However, if faced with a request for PND clinicians have two options: they could either be led by patient autonomy and therefore respond to patient requests for PND for deafness with selective TOP for the 'wrong' hearing status, or they could decide that they would not offer tests for certain conditions. Deafness is an interesting condition since it cannot be obviously defined as 'serious' in the way that Huntington's Disease might be, or 'non-serious' as colour blindness could be perceived. Different people have varying perspectives on the impact of deafness.

Some deaf parents have said they will not seek genetic counselling because they worry that they will be told not to have children (Israel, 1995). This should not happen within the present context of genetic counselling as indicated above. The focus of genetic counselling for deafness is no longer on prevention of deafness but rather on the individual needs of patients and their families (Arnos et al., 1992).

There is often the misconception that the aim of genetic counselling is to prevent genetic disorders. Das (1996) states that:

> The high incidence of genetic causes [of deafness] indicates that steps should be taken to facilitate genetic counselling and conceivably to reduce the numbers affected.

It is often this kind of misinformation that fuels arguments from Deaf activists that genetic counselling aims to destroy the Deaf community (by reducing the numbers of babies born with deafness, which will ultimately mean that the adult Deaf community will gradually decline). A discussion of Deaf cultural attitudes towards genetics is given in more detail in later sections.

Potential outcomes of the genetic research

The results of molecular genetic research will provide a more specific genetic counselling service to families with deafness. For families who test positive, for example for a specific recessive gene fault that could cause deafness, it would be possible to identify whether hearing parents or siblings were carriers of such a gene fault and to offer more specific information about the chances of having deaf children. Genetic testing could also offer a quick and early diagnosis of deafness in a newborn baby, in addition to the audiological testing that is currently be available.

Gene therapy could replace the need for cochlear implants, and the obvious pain and risks that major surgery brings. It has also been suggested that, in the first half of the twenty-first century, genetic research will have solved the problem of regenerating missing or malformed hair cells in the cochlea (Wheeler, 1998).

The outcome of genetic research on families with deafness is summarized by Arnos et al. (1992):

Advances in molecular genetics will eventually bring about new options for prenatal diagnosis of deafness and prenatal or postnatal treatment. Deaf and hard-of-hearing people and parents of deaf children will surely have different feelings and may make different choices regarding the options that will be available to them. . . . Some of the issues that arise may be similar to those that have come up as genetic technology has been applied to the diagnosis and treatment of other hereditary conditions. The sociocultural aspects of deafness will lend additional considerations to these discussions.

Deafness and the family

Communication

There are many different communication methods open to deaf people: for example, sign language such as British Sign Language (BSL) or Sign Supported English (SSE), gesture, speech, lip-reading, finger spelling and writing. Signed language can be unique languages in their own right, having a distinct grammar and structure that are different from spoken language.

Research has shown a relationship between lack of communication and a deficit in subsequent cognitive development. This is described by Oliver Sacks in his book *Seeing Voices* (1990):

> . . . if communication goes awry, it will affect intellectual growth, social inter-course, language development, and emotional attitudes, all at once, simultane-ously and inseparably. And this . . . is what may happen when a child is born deaf.

After a diagnosis has been made, the subsequent choice of communication route is very important since it will impact enormously on the eventual functioning of the family as a whole (Kluwin and Gaustad, 1991). The research of Kluwin and Gaustad showed that parents made decisions about the means of communication based on the level of deafness and availability of local services. Interestingly, an association was found between the level of education of the mother and willingness to learn sign language, and therefore a subsequent choice of signing communication for the deaf child.

Hearing parents of deaf children

Ninety per cent of deaf children have hearing parents (CADS, 1987). For parents with no family history of deafness, having a child who is unexpectedly deaf is sometimes perceived in the same way as other congenital genetic conditions would be, i.e. as a handicap (Mindel and Feldman, 1987; Schein, 1989; Koester and Meadow-Orlans, 1990; Luterman and Ross, 1991). The reason for this may be because the image of having a 'normal' child has been shattered. Parents may go through a grief process as they mourn the loss of the potential child they had been expecting (Sloman et al., 1993); they may also worry about how they will bring up their child and how they will communicate (Atkins,

1994). Most parents want to know what caused the deafness in their child(ren) (Vernon and Andrews, 1990). It is therefore understandable that hearing parents might want to utilize genetic technology to determine the hearing status of a child before it is born, and may prefer to have hearing children.

Deaf children tend to have more behavioural problems than hearing children (Meadow, 1976). According to research accumulated by Schum (1991) deaf children are sometimes described as being 'impulsive, rigid, immature, egocentric, displaying an absence of inner controls and empathy, and having a limited self-awareness'. However, as also reported in the above research, deaf children of deaf parents are less likely to have the above characteristics than deaf children of hearing parents. This indicates that hearing parents have more problems coping with deaf children than deaf parents (this is discussed further in Chapter 5).

Deaf parents of deaf children

Approximately 85–90% of deaf individuals marry another deaf person (this statistic does not encompass individuals with late-onset or old age deafness) (Schein, 1989) and 90% of deaf parents have hearing children (Israel, 1995). Therefore, 10% of deaf parents have deaf children. The birth of a child with unexpected hearing status, which could be deaf or hearing depending on what the deaf parents were hoping for, can evoke a similar reaction to that of hearing parents with the birth of a deaf child (Schein, 1989).

Deaf parents understand the way of life for a deaf person and know what to expect with regard to education and communication, more so than hearing parents might (Meadow-Orlans, 1990). Some deaf parents may therefore prefer to have a deaf child, who will fit into their social network and culture and use the same communication methods they do (Jordan, 1991). Dolnick (1993) comments on this in *Deafness as Culture*: 'So strong is the feeling of cultural solidarity that many deaf parents cheer on discovering that their baby is deaf.'

For some Deaf people, having a deaf child would ensure that the Deaf community's communication tools and culture are maintained for another generation. Making this ideal a reality could technically be possible with the use of genetic technology, i.e. through the use of PND and selective TOP of a hearing fetus. Other deaf parents may not want their child to go through the same obstacles of being deaf in a hearing world that they went through, and so would prefer to have a hearing child.

Deafness and the community

The deaf community

The **deaf community** (lower-case d) is a term used to describe a group of people, including deaf children and adults, hard-of-hearing, hearing-impaired and deafened individuals, hearing family members such as hearing children of deaf parents and hearing parents of deaf children as well as interpreters (Israel, 1995). This community involves all people where deafness has had an impact and individuals use a variety of communication methods, such as speech, BSL or SSE.

The **Deaf community** (upper-case D) is a smaller section of the main deaf community and refers to people who are culturally Deaf, who tend to have profound, prelingual deafness, and who use sign language (e.g. BSL not SSE) as the primary or preferred method of communication (Padden, 1980; Christiansen, 1991).

Sociological vs medical model of deafness

The culturally Deaf view deafness from the cultural or sociological perspective, i.e. that deafness is a condition to be understood and preserved, as opposed to the medical perspective, often adopted by hearing parents, medical professionals and the hearing world, who may see deafness as a pathology to be treated or cured. The culture binds Deaf people together with common values, social customs, history and experiences (Arnos, Israel, and Cunningham, 1991).

The medical model of deafness emphasizes that deafness is an impairment, whereas the sociological model does not see deafness as an impairment, but rather focuses on social arrangements and group characteristics (Christiansen, 1991). Therefore, according to this model deafness is not simply the opposite of hearing, but offers an enriched opportunity to live a full, productive life as part of a unique community, sharing common perspectives and goals (Jordan, 1991):

> Deaf people have always rejected the notion that they are defective or dysfunctional and, thus, have resented the focus on prevention and cure at the expense of more attention to better services and enhancement of the lives of people who are deaf.

Many individuals in the Deaf community see themselves more as part of an 'ethnic minority' group rather than as members of the disabled community (Johnson and Erting, 1989). The sociological model of deafness views society's beliefs as being the driving force in making deaf people handicapped. For example, some deaf people cannot use the telephone without special modifications to allow them to do so; these difficulties do not arise because the person is deaf but because society has determined that telephones are mainly accessible to hearing people, so enforcing discrimination against deaf people.

Attitudes from the hearing world can be a driving force in discrimination:

> Negative attitudes towards deafness held by hearing people may act as real barriers to the success of deaf persons seeking employment, educational opportunity, or interpersonal relationships (Schroedel and Schiff, 1972).

Medical professionals working with deaf families need to be aware of the sociological as well as the medical perspectives of deafness, since they will see patients who utilize the different approaches. Having such an awareness means that terminology can be adapted so as not to cause offence. For example, within the clinical genetics service, if a professional is aware that a deaf patient does not see having a deaf child as a problem, then it would be insensitive to talk to them in terms of there being a 'risk' of having a deaf child or else referring to deafness as 'abnormal' and hearing as 'normal' within the genetic counselling process. Instead professionals would talk about the 'chance' of having a deaf child and use the terms 'deafness' and 'hearing' as they are without saying either is 'abnormal'.

Terminology

Professionals, researchers and individuals affected by hearing loss use different terminology to describe similar concepts, and this can cause considerable confusion (Grundfast and Rosen, 1992). At the European Hereditary Deafness Concerted Action Conference in Milan 1996, Stephens stated that the medical term 'deafness' should be avoided since it had many different meanings in different contexts. Instead, he suggested 'hearing impairment' should be used to cover all aspects of hearing loss. The given definition of hearing impairment was:

> Defective function of the auditory system which may be measured using psycho-acoustical or physiological techniques (Stephens, 1996).

However, the importance of the term 'hearing impaired' is questioned by social science and genetic counselling researchers such as Israel (1995) who point out that some deaf people do not like the idea that being without hearing makes them defective or 'impaired' in some way. To such people being deaf is a positive experience and being labelled as hearing impaired is something they may not receive positively.

Through conducting this research I discovered that the term 'hearing impaired' was used infrequently by the participants. Generally speaking, most of those who called themselves 'hard-of-hearing', 'hearing-impaired' or 'deafened' tended to associate with the hearing world and used oral communication. Of those who called themselves 'deaf', some used oral communication and some sign language. Many such deaf sign-language users associated with the Deaf community.

For ease of reading, in this chapter the term 'deafness' is used to refer to any level of hearing loss.

Attitudes towards medical intervention

Deaf and hearing people often have different views and beliefs about medical intervention for deafness, primarily because deafness can be viewed from different perspectives. Many culturally Deaf people are sensitive to threats to their community; this reaction has been clearly demonstrated in the resistance to cochlear implants (Gibson, 1991). Deaf adults may think that deaf children should be put through extensive surgery to try to make them hearing when they do not perceive being deaf as a problem.

There is a fear that the use of genetic technology will reduce the numbers of deaf children being born, so having a direct effect on the viability of the Deaf community (Grundfast and Rosen, 1992; Middleton, Hewison and Mueller, 1998). This fear of genetic research is deep-rooted in Deaf culture, primarily because of the appalling way deaf people have been treated throughout history, often in the name of eugenics (Bahan, 1989) (see Chapter 1).

Wheeler, from the Deafness Research Foundation in the USA, believes that research into finding cures for deafness is still compatible with the preservation of the Deaf community (Wheeler, 1998). He suggests that by removing communication barriers so that sign-language users have equal access to 'learning and enjoyment of life', a better quality of life will be achieved. At the same time, those who wish to use treatments or cures can do so. However, Wheeler does not acknowledge the real argument from many culturally Deaf people: that since most deaf children are born into hearing families, decisions to have treatments or cures will be made by hearing people who probably are not aware of the cultural model of deafness. Hearing people, with their affinity to the hearing world and ignorance of the Deaf world, will make decisions for their deaf child according to their 'hearing' perspective. Therefore, deaf children may be offered a cure for their deafness before they are old enough to make choices for themselves, so missing the opportunity to be part of a community they could naturally belong to.

Many Deaf people aim to educate hearing people into having an awareness of the Deaf community so that parents are better informed about the options open to their deaf child. However, input from deaf people about the medical or educational management of deafness has largely been ignored in the past (Lane, 1984). There needs to be a working partnership between parents of deaf children, the Deaf community and professionals working in deafness to ensure services for all deaf people are improved (Mohay, 1991).

The British Deaf Association has created a policy on genetics (BDA 2003) which 'demands' that all genetic counsellors in the UK receive deaf awareness training so that they become familiar with Deaf attitudes.

Attitudes towards genetic testing

Several other studies have looked at attitudes of deaf and hearing people towards genetic testing for deafness. Middleton, Hewison and Mueller (1998) documented the views of 87 deaf participants who mainly identified with the

Deaf culture. This study showed a very negative attitude towards genetics and fear that genetic technology would be used in some way to destroy the Deaf community. This study also showed that there was a small group of Deaf participants who wanted to have prenatal testing for deafness and also preferred to have deaf children. There was the theoretical possibility that they may actually choose to have a TOP for a hearing fetus. The same authors conducted a much larger study documenting the views of 644 deaf individuals, 143 hard-of-hearing individuals and 527 hearing individuals with either a deaf parent or a deaf child (Middleton, Hewison and Mueller, 2001; Middleton, 2004). Here participants were collected from medical and education sources, social services, charities and support groups for the deaf. From this study, 49% of hearing participants with a family history of deafness, 39% of hard-of-hearing and deafened participants and 21% of deaf participants said they would all be interested in having PND for deafness, with 16% of hearing, 11% of hard-of-hearing and deafened, and 5% of deaf participants interested in TOP for deafness. Therefore, in all groups, the majority said they would only use PND for preparation, rather than because they wanted to have a TOP of a deaf fetus. Furthermore 3 deaf individuals (2%) said they would consider having PND with selective TOP of a hearing fetus since they preferred to have deaf children (Middleton, Hewison and Mueller, 2001; Middleton, 2004). Other studies documenting such attitudes have not demonstrated such extreme views (for example, see Brunger et al., 2000; Dagan et al., 2002; Stern et al., 2002; Martinez et al., 2003).

The study described below aims to add to the literature on this subject by examining the attitudes of a large group of deaf and hearing parents of deaf children. It could be argued that the issue of PND for deafness is actually of the most relevance to parents who have already had deaf children, since this is an obvious group for whom PND services are currently available.

Methods

Participants

A large sample of participants was collected, a subset of whom were parents of deaf children. In the sample as a whole, including parents and non-parents, 644 were deaf, 143 were hard-of-hearing or deafened, and 527 were hearing individuals with either a deaf parent or a deaf child. The hearing status classifications were made according to how the participants viewed their situation. For example, if a participant called themselves 'hard-of-hearing' this tended to mean that they had a mild or moderate hearing loss; if they were 'deafened' then this usually meant they had lost their hearing later on in life. Sociodemographic data relating to these participants has been published elsewhere (Middleton, Hewison and Mueller, 2001; Middleton, 1999, 2004). Some of the results are analysed for cultural affinity, i.e. from a Deaf sense. Culturally Deaf participants were those who considered themselves deaf, hard-of-hearing or deafened, who said BSL was their preferred language and who mixed more in the Deaf community than in the hearing world. A subset of this population, who were parents of deaf children, was selected for representation in the present chapter. Such participants had one or more deaf children and, of these parents, 74 were deaf, 34 were hard-of-hearing or deafened, and 432 were hearing.

Ascertainment

Ascertainment for the study occurred in the UK between June 1998 and June 1999. Twenty-eight different methods were used to collect the study sample, including various hospital departments such as genetics, ENT, audiology, social services for the deaf, schools, colleges, charities, deaf clubs and deaf conferences. A letter was sent to each health or education professional involved with the potential study participants, asking if they could pass on a questionnaire to their clients. Participants who used sign language as their preferred language were given the option of completing the questionnaire via a sign language interpreter. The questionnaire was also sent out to subscribers of three different magazines for deaf people. Ethical approval was granted for the study by St James's University Hospital Ethics Committee, Leeds.

Questionnaire

The study questionnaire was designed to be as Deaf-sensitive as possible, with support from Deaf facilitators who checked how easy it would be to translate into BSL. There were some words that had to be changed, e.g. the term 'abortion' was used rather than 'termination of pregnancy' since this translated more fluently into BSL.

There was a total of 32 questions, a selection of which are discussed in this chapter. They covered issues surrounding preference for having deaf or hearing children, interest in utilizing a test in pregnancy for deafness, reasons for having PND for deafness and interest in TOP for deafness and 'hearingness' (i.e. ending the pregnancy if the fetus is found not to have the deafness-causing gene faults, since the parents prefer to have deaf children). Results relating to these questions have already been published elsewhere for the large ascertained study sample (Middleton, 1999, 2004; Middleton, Hewison and Mueller, 2001). Additional issues relating only to parents of deaf children are published for the first time in this chapter. These cover attitudes towards PND for a range of conditions, success of communication with deaf children, assessment of level of support received after obtaining diagnosis of deafness in child, views on advantage or disadvantage of deafness, burden of deafness, wish for a cure for deafness, success of obtaining a diagnosis and success of obtaining education for deaf child(ren).

Results

Responses from deaf and hard-of-hearing/deafened participants followed the same patterns and so have been grouped together and labelled as 'deaf'. The actual level of hearing loss that these participants had varied from mild through to profound. Again, for more detailed figures, statistics and raw data see Middleton (1999, 2004); Middleton, Hewison and Mueller (2001).

There was a significant association between hearing status of the parents and the number of deaf children they had (χ^2 = 16.1, df = 2, p < 0.001). Deaf parents were more likely than hearing parents to have 3 or 4 deaf children, whereas hearing parents were the most likely to have 2 deaf children.

There was a significant association between hearing status of the parents and preference for having deaf or hearing children (Table 2.1). Most hearing parents preferred to have hearing children; most deaf parents did not mind the hearing status of future children. This result, together with all subsequent results shown here, follows the same pattern for the whole sample (Middleton, 1999, 2003; Middleton, Hewison and Mueller, 2001).There was a significant association between hearing status of the parents and PND for deafness (Table 2.2). Deaf participants were more likely to say no to PND for deafness, and hearing participants were more likely to say yes. Of the deaf parents interested in PND for deafness, six (19%) were culturally Deaf and the rest were non-culturally deaf.

Reasons for having PND for deafness

Of the deaf parents and hearing parents who would have PND for deafness, the highest proportion for each group would do so just to prepare personally for the child's needs (Table 2.1).

Attitudes towards termination of pregnancy for the 'wrong' hearing status

There was a significant association between hearing status of the parents and attitudes towards TOP for deafness (Table 2.1). Eight per cent of hearing parents and 1% of deaf parents said they would consider having a TOP for deafness. In the remainder of the sample deaf parents were more likely to think TOP for deafness should be illegal, whereas hearing parents were more likely than deaf parents to think it should be available.

Table 2.1. Summary of selected results

Selected answers	Participants		
	Deaf parents	Hearing parents	Statistics
Would prefer to have deaf children	12/105 (11%)	2/417 (0%)	
Would prefer to have hearing children	31/105 (30%)	286/417 (69%)	$\chi^2 = 31$, d.f. = 1, $p < 0.001$
Don't mind the hearing status of future children	61/105 (58%)	120/417 (29%)	
Yes to test in pregnancy for deafness	32/108 (30%)	229/430 (53%)	$\chi^2 = 20.5$, d.f. = 2, $p < 0.001$
No to test in pregnancy for deafness	61/108 (56%)	150/430 (35%)	
Test in pregnancy could prepare for language needs of child	22/32 (69%)	160/229 (70%)	
Test in pregnancy could offer personal preparation for the child	27/32 (84%)	199/229 (87%)	Statistical analysis not applicable
Test in pregnancy would avoid putting my child through unnecessary medical tests	16/32 (50%)	109/229(48%)	
Would consider having abortion if fetus is deaf	1/96 (1%)	32/412 (8%)	$\chi^2 = 9.8$, d.f. = 1, $p = 0.002$
Think abortion for deafness should be illegal	69/96 (72%)	224/412 (54%)	
Would consider having abortion if fetus is hearing	0/94 (0%)	0/400 (0%)	Statistical analysis not applicable
Think abortion for a hearing fetus should be illegal	77/94 (82%)	315/400 (79%)	

Numbers in brackets denote approximate percentages.
As only selected data is presented some totals are incomplete. There are also some missing responses to certain questions.

There was no significant association between hearing status of the parents and attitudes towards TOP for 'hearingness', i.e. a hearing fetus when a deaf baby is preferred (Table 2.1). No parents were interested in this, and in both groups the majority thought it should be illegal.

Table 2.2. Gradient of conditions for which hearing and deaf parents of deaf children would consider a TOP

Percentage of participants who would consider an abortion for each condition					
Hearing parents					
0% Hearingness Wrong sex	1% Treatable physical defect, e.g. cleft palate	8% Deafness	11% Severe painful disorder, starting age 40, incurable	19% Blindness	57% Severe, genetic disorder leading to death age 5
Deaf parents					
0% Hearingness Wrong sex	1% Deafness	3% Treatable physical defect, e.g. cleft palate	6% Severe painful disorder, starting age 40, incurable [Huntington's Disease]	14% Blindness	58% Severe, genetic disorder leading to death age 5 [Tay Sachs Disease]

Communication

There was a significant association between hearing status of the parents and success of communication with the deaf child (χ^2 = 40.6, d.f. = 2, p < 0.001) (Figure 2.1). Deaf parents were much more likely to be 'very successful' at communicating with their deaf children whereas hearing parents were more likely to just be 'successful' or 'OK' at communication.

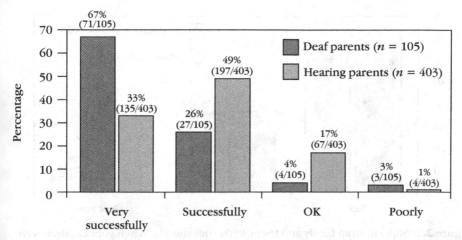

Figure 2.1. Success of communication with deaf child. The question is 'How successfully do you manage to communicate with your deaf child(ren) (in speech, sign language or other forms)?'

Comments from parents who said the communication between parent and child was successful

'Using BSL as a first language in the home and then spoken English gives solid foundations for communicating as a family.' [Hearing parent of deaf children]

'[Communication with deaf children is successful] because we all use BSL since I come from a large deaf family where no communication is a problem.' [Deaf parent of deaf children]

'One child is oral and one uses BSL. As the latter grows, our fluency in sign is becoming insufficient for the complexity of his communication. I use ANY means I can from speech, sign, mime, role-playing, drawing – whatever.' [Hearing parent of deaf children]

Comments from parents who said the communication between parent and child was OK or poor

'All our arguments are triggered by communication difficulties.' [Hard-of-hearing parent of deaf children]

'[communication is] frustrating sometimes getting worse.' [Hearing parent of deaf children]

Assessment of support

There was a significant association between hearing status of the parents and the feeling that support was received from family and friends at the time of the diagnosis of deafness in the child ($\chi^2 = 10$, d.f. = 2, $p = 0.006$) (Figure 2.2). Deaf parents were more likely than hearing parents to feel that they received support from family and friends.

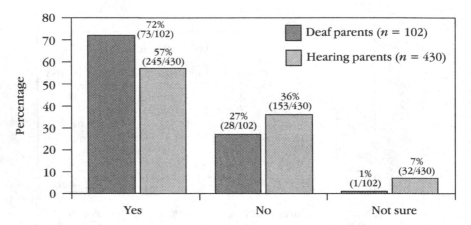

Figure 2.2. Support from family and friends. The question is 'When your children were diagnosed as deaf, did you feel you received enough support from family and friends?'.

There was no difference between the hearing status of the parents and feelings that enough support was received from health professionals (Figure 2.3). Approximately equal numbers of both deaf and hearing parents said they did and did not receive enough support from health professionals.

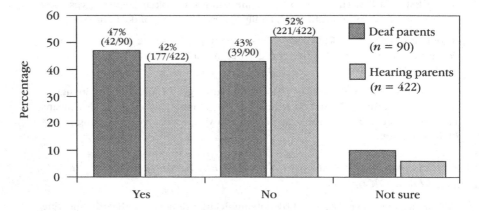

Figure 2.3. Support from health professionals. The question is 'When your children were diagnosed as deaf, did you feel you received enough support from health professionals?'.

Comments from parents who did not receive enough support from family and friends

'Family were confused. Isolation was worst aspect as friends drifted away – some didn't want their children picking up funny voice noises, some believed deaf children are violent.' [Hearing parent of deaf children]

'As family and friends had never seen a deaf child before, I think they were frightened.' [Hearing parent of deaf children]

Comments from parents who did not receive enough support from health professionals

'Being deaf myself I did not feel I required extra emotional support but must admit I had my own way of dealing with things and didn't always see eye to eye with the so called health professionals.' [Deaf parent of deaf children]

'Health professionals thought we were disappointed that he was born deaf – they even suggested an operation to help him hear!! Of course we refused.' [Culturally Deaf parent of deaf children]

'We have found health professionals to be sadly lacking in knowledge of hearing loss – some desperately ignorant. Medical staff are probably the worst offenders – without understanding, it is impossible to be supportive.' [Hearing parent of deaf children]

'Health professionals were particularly unhelpful as they saw it in purely medical terms.' [Hearing parent of deaf children]

'No doctors, only technicians available, therefore little information, no-one to talk to about the deafness. Poor staffing problems. No home visits to see how getting on. There should be more deaf awareness.' [Hearing parent of deaf children]

Comment from parents who did not need support

'Deaf myself; didn't need support, everyone else needed support to accept it.' [Deaf parent of deaf children]

Comment from parents who felt they were supported

'Health professionals excellent in their support. Family thrown into a disability they did not understand how to relate to or understand.' [Hearing parent of deaf children]

Impact of deafness on child and family

There was a significant association between the hearing status of the parents and feelings about whether the deaf children were advantaged or disadvantaged because of their deafness ($\chi^2 = 58.1$, d.f. = 2, $p < 0.001$) (Figure 2.4). Hearing parents were more likely to think their deaf child was disadvantaged while deaf parents thought their child was both advantaged and disadvantaged.

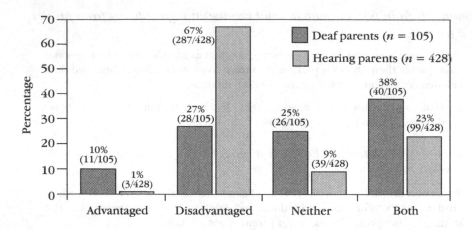

Figure 2.4. Advantage or disadvantage of deafness in children. The question is 'Do you feel that your children are advantaged or disadvantaged in any way because of their hearing loss?'.

Comments from parents who thought that deafness for their child was an advantage

'I could share my skills and knowledge of deafness. I could understand her needs better. Lots of people confused me by trying to control our situations.' [Deaf parent of deaf children]

'At home we're all deaf family so they never felt "left out". It's society without "deaf awareness" that made them feel disadvantaged! Otherwise we are all happy and close knit family with same rich language, culture.' [Culturally Deaf parent of deaf children]

'Being deaf myself the children were advantaged as I knew what the problems were and knew what to do.' [Deaf parent of deaf children]

Comments from parents who thought deafness for their child was a disadvantage

'He misses out on conversation and information going on around him. Both he and his brother are disadvantaged in play and general children's chit chat. This disadvantage would be eased in the home if support were given at the earliest moment with language.' [Hearing parent of deaf children]

'Communication is a major problem, especially because most people make no effort to understand deaf issues.' [Hearing parent of deaf children]

'They sometimes feel very restricted and lonely because of their hearing loss.' [Hearing parent of deaf children]

Comments from one parent who thought deafness for their child was both an advantage and a disadvantage

'Advantaged in deaf world/family. Disadvantaged in hearing world (occasionally).'
[Culturally Deaf parent of deaf children]

There was a significant association between hearing status of the parents and actual burden of deafness ($\chi^2 = 30.5$, d.f. = 3, $p < 0.001$) (Figure 2.5). Deaf parents were more likely to say that deafness caused no burden whereas hearing participants were more likely to say that it caused a level of burden ranging from a little to very great.

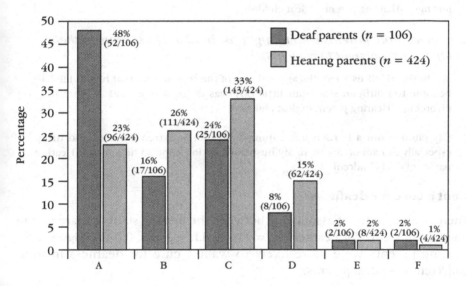

Figure 2.5. Burden of deafness. The question is: 'Please can you say whether you feel an actual burden of having a child who is deaf.' (A) Deafness in my child(ren) causes no burden to me. (B) Deafness in my child(ren) causes very little burden to me. (C) The burden is moderately great, but I can cope with it. (D) The burden is very great but I can cope with it. (E) The burden is too great and I have difficulty coping with it. (F) I'm not sure.

Comments from parents who thought that deafness in their children caused no burden

'As we are deaf too having a deaf son was a joy - relationships are strong and continue in adulthood because he has deaf friends too - so we all integrate socially. [Culturally Deaf parent of deaf children]

'It is hard work and one has to try and remain positive. The burden is not my deaf child - trying to access the right education, speech therapy and all the family trying to learn a new language without support is the burden. It costs money to learn BSL' [Hearing parent of deaf children]

Comments from parents who thought there was some burden of having a child with deafness

'The struggle for education rights and support were a burden of stress and anxiety during her school years. In itself deafness isn't a burden, but the discrimination against my child's human rights and the suffering this caused was heartbreaking at times.' [Deaf parent of deaf children]

'I think this varied with the age of the child. It is harder to cope when they are younger as you also have to deal with your own and the extended family's feelings.' [Hearing parent of deaf children]

Comments from parents who thought the burden of deafness in their children was too great to cope with

'My husband left us 3 months ago and one of the reasons was that he felt life had become too difficult since our little boy was diagnosed as deaf. We are now divorcing.' [Hearing parent of deaf children]

'My child is not a burden but coping with him is extremely hard and tiring especially as I am on my own. My husband couldn't cope so he left us.' [Hearing parent of deaf children]

Want a cure for deafness?

There was a significant association between the hearing status of parents and opinion on a cure for deafness ($\chi^2 = 116.4$, d.f. = 2, $p < 0.001$) (Figure 2.6). Hearing parents were more likely to want a cure for deafness in their child(ren) than deaf parents.

Comments from parents who would like a cure for the deaf child

'My eldest son desperately wants to be a hearing child and listen to music and know what they are saying like other children his age.' [Hearing parent of deaf child]

'To hear would be a bonus, but not essential.' [Deaf parent of deaf child]

Comments from parents who would not like a cure for their deaf child

'I wish both my children were deaf even though this is probably very selfish and I never tell them that.' [Deaf parent of one deaf and one hearing child]

'Deaf culture is his life – he's happy and well adjusted, responsible and leads a fulfilling life.' [Hearing parent of deaf child]

'As he's very happy child and full of confidence – I even asked him if he want to hear – he said NO!' [Culturally Deaf parent of deaf child]

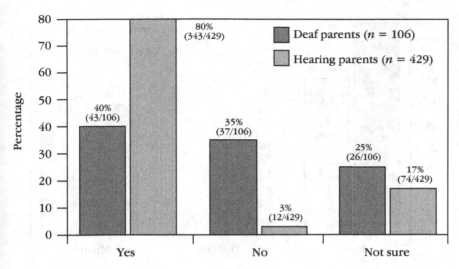

Figure 2.6. Cure for deafness. The question was 'If there was a cure or treatment for deafness, would you want your children to have it?'.

'I wouldn't dream of forcing hearing children to become deaf by giving treatment to become deaf so you can imagine how deaf child feels with all medicine's view trying to cure him or her, thus giving child's feelings into low self-esteem.' [Culturally Deaf parent of deaf children]

Experience of gaining a diagnosis

There was a significant association between hearing status and experience of obtaining a diagnosis (χ^2 = 9.1, d.f. = 2, p = 0.01) (Figure 2.7). Deaf parents were more likely to think the experience of obtaining a diagnosis of deafness in their child was 'easy and straightforward', whereas hearing parents were more likely than deaf parents to think it was 'difficult or complicated'.

Comments from parents who said the process was easy

'We knew our daughter is deaf before the medical diagnosis. It was easy to accept the fact when it was officially diagnosed.' [Culturally Deaf parent of deaf children]

'The problem was found very quickly. Referrals were made quickly and smoothly although the news was painful.' [Hearing parent of deaf children]

Comments from parents who said the process was a mixture of easy and difficult experiences

'Difficult experience with my first child. Easy, straightforward experience with my second child.' [Deaf parent of deaf children]

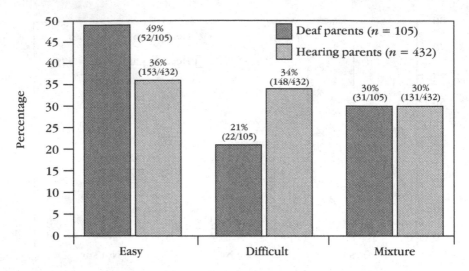

Figure 2.7. Experience of gaining a diagnosis. The question was 'Please say how you found the experience of obtaining a diagnosis for your deaf child (easy and straightforward, difficult or complicated or a mixture of these experiences)'.

Comments from parents who said the process was difficult

'It was a battle. I suspected deafness at 4 mths, but was ignored, told I had postnatal depression and that my son had normal hearing. After phone calls and visits to clinics, he was diagnosed at 1yr 10mths.' [Hearing parent of deaf child]

'Had to take child to hospital about 6 times to convince them he had a hearing loss. Eventually, I sent my husband with him and toys, etc. he couldn't hear and they then agreed. He should have had aids from 1 yr – not 3!' [Hearing parent of deaf child]

'It was a protracted/anxious drawn out process almost a year before a proper diagnosis was given. Appointment delays, equipment broken, bureaucracy, etc, etc.' [Hearing parent of deaf child]

'We had enormous difficulty in persuading GPs that our son was deaf. Visits to specialists were brief, unsatisfactory and horribly patronizing. I dreaded them.' [Hearing parent of deaf children]

Experience of gaining education

There was no significant association between hearing status of the parents and experience of gaining educational provision for the deaf child (Figure 2.8). Approximately the same numbers of deaf and hearing parents found the experience easy and difficult.

A selection of comments from parents about the experience of obtaining education for their children follows.

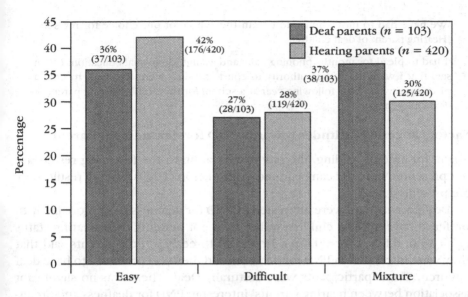

Figure 2.8. Experience of gaining educational provision. The question was 'Please say how you found the experience of obtaining educational provision for your deaf child (easy and straightforward, difficult or complicated or a mixture of these experiences)'.

Comments from parents who thought the process was easy

'We had no problem with educational provision as we had our experience at deaf school while we were younger.' [Culturally Deaf parent of deaf children]

'Thankfully we are in a very good area. Everybody was more than helpful in sorting out the children's education.' [Hearing parent of deaf children]

Comments from parents who thought the process was a mixture of easy and difficult experiences

'Only because his mother and I understand the system, I fought our local authority and won. It would and has been extremely difficult for many parents.' [Hearing parent of deaf children]

'Authorities without knowledge of deaf culture, language and communities shouldn't place deaf child into mainstream schools without parents' needs to access other choices of excellent deaf school. It's always money problem with authority.' [Culturally Deaf parent of deaf children; text translated from sign language by participant]

Comments from parents who thought the process was difficult

'Still unresolved. We're going to tribunal at present moment. Most support he has received we have had to instigate. School's medical officer has been very supportive but LEA not and have opposed us over use of BSL.'[Hearing parent of deaf children]

'We have had to move house to obtain the school of our choice for my son.' [Hearing parent of deaf children]

'I had to plead for months phoning daily and asking for special education. I then said that I would take the authority to court and they were then able to fund a place for my child the following year at a school for the deaf.' [Hearing parent of deaf children]

Factors affecting attitudes towards PND for deafness for parents

Again, for ease of reading, the raw data relating to the following results are not presented here but can be found in Middleton (1999). Overall results only are presented here.

Deaf parents who were interested in PND for deafness were more likely to prefer to have hearing children rather than not minding their hearing status ($\chi^2 = 15.6$, d.f. = 1, $p < 0.001$). However, three (9%) deaf parents said that they were interested in PND for deafness and they also preferred to have deaf children. These participants were culturally Deaf. There was no significant association between hearing parents' interest in PND for deafness and preference for having hearing children. This was because most hearing parents preferred to have hearing children.

There was no significant association between parents' interest in PND and their opinion on TOP for deafness, number of deaf children they had, their assessment of support for their deaf children and their experience of obtaining a diagnosis.

Attitudes towards PND for deafness vs success of communication

If the whole group of all parents is considered together, the association between interest in PND for deafness and success of communication is significant ($\chi^2 = 9.8$, d.f. = 4, $p = 0.04$). Parents who were interested in PND for deafness said the communication with their child ranged from successful to poor (i.e. not 'very successful'). Therefore, presence of less than perfect communication with a deaf child is directly linked to parental interest in having PND for deafness (with the preference for having deaf children).

Attitudes towards PND for deafness vs impact of deafness

There was a small but significant association between deaf parents' interest in PND for deafness and their opinion on whether their children are advantaged or disadvantaged ($\chi^2 = 6.0$, d.f. = 2, $p = 0.05$). Deaf parents interested in PND for deafness were more likely to think their child was disadvantaged by deafness. There was no association between hearing parents' interest in PND for deafness and opinion on whether their children were advantaged or disadvantaged. As shown previously, most hearing parents thought their child was disadvantaged by their deafness.

Deaf parents who were interested in PND for deafness were more likely to think there was some degree of burden associated with having a deaf child (χ^2 = 5.1, d.f. = 1, p = 0.02). There was no association between hearing parents' interest in PND for deafness and opinion on the burden of deafness. Most hearing parents saw the deafness in their child as a burden to the child.

Attitudes towards PND for deafness vs wanting a cure for deafness

Deaf parents interested in PND for deafness were the most likely to want a cure for deafness for their child (χ^2 = 8.6, d.f. = 2, p = 0.01). There was no association between hearing parents' interest in PND for deafness and wanting a cure for deafness. As shown previously, most hearing parents wanted a cure for their deaf child.

Attitudes towards PND for deafness is experience of gaining education

There was some association between parents' attitudes towards PND for deafness and their opinion on the experience of gaining education. Hearing parents who were interested in PND for deafness found the experience of obtaining education for their deaf child difficult and complicated (not significant, but slight association demonstrated χ^2 = 10.9, d.f. = 4, p = 0.03).

Discussion

The aim of this research was to determine attitudes towards genetic testing for deafness, so that information could be provided to help improve clinical services offered to deaf families. By gaining more of an understanding of how people feel about utilizing the technologies available to them it is possible to plan for the potential uptake of testing within clinical genetics services. The following extract provides a brief summary of why the current research is important:

> The new human genetics is a fast-moving field. Its development raises many questions concerning policies for clinical practice, such as who should be offered genetic services, what services should comprise, and how decisions concerning these matters should be made. Discussions about the effects and desired scope of genetic developments in the UK are held between scientists, clinicians and ethicists, but seldom do they involve the general public. Ignoring public opinion in this way runs the risk that services may be developed which do not meet people's needs optimally, and which may result in social and psychological harm (Michie et al., 1995).

Genetic counselling in general could be improved by more insight into the particular concerns and fears of patients with different disabilities. Past research has looked at lay understanding of genetics (Chapple, May, and Campion, 1995; Richards, 1997) and at case-study discussion of issues relevant to patients with certain genetic conditions (Marteau and Richards, 1996). However, more research is needed to fully explore particular concerns that are relevant to patients with specific genetic conditions. This is addressed by the current research, which demonstrates how deafness impacts on the individual and their family.

Study sample

A total of 540 questionnaires were received from parents of deaf children. This sample is much larger than other studies documenting the attitudes of parents towards genetic testing for conditions other than deafness (e.g. Kaback et al., 1984; Wertz et al., 1991; Green, 1992; Sagi, Shiloh and Cohen, 1992; Watson et al., 1992b). It is also larger than the other studies involving deaf adults and hearing parents of deaf children (e.g. Brunger et al., 2000; Dagan et al., 2002; Stern et al., 2002; Martinez et al., 2003).

Most parents in the study had two profoundly deaf children who were between 10 and 20 years old. Therefore, such parents would have knowledge and experience of the greatest level of hearing loss with all the complications associated with this. Also, because the children were in the 10–20 age bracket, parents would have had time to get used to the deafness in their children, more so than parents of newly diagnosed children. This could mean that their opinions about deafness were more consistent and established than someone who was just starting to deal with deafness in their child.

There were more hearing parents of deaf children than deaf parents of deaf children. This reflects the ascertainment procedures employed (hearing participants who were targeted tended to already be parents), but also because of the fact that deaf children are more likely to have hearing parents (CADS, 1987).

Issues surrounding PND for deafness

Preference for having deaf or hearing children

Most deaf parents did not mind the hearing status of future children; most hearing participants preferred to have hearing children. This implies that deaf parents are flexible about coping with either a deaf or a hearing child, or perhaps they had greater awareness of what deafness in a child would mean and therefore able to accept this more readily than someone with no personal experience of it. Some of this sample of deaf parents were culturally Deaf and if so may have preferred to have deaf children so that they could pass on their language, history and culture to the next generation, thus keeping the Deaf community alive.

Attitudes towards PND for deafness

Hearing participants were more likely (53%) to be interested in using PND for deafness than deaf participants (30%). This pattern fits in with results from the larger study already published (Middleton, Hewison and Mueller, 2001; Middleton, 2004) and also with results from another study done in the USA which used the same study questionnaire (Stern et al., 2002). This implies that deafness in the next child is of greater interest to hearing parents than it is to deaf parents, presumably because deafness is seen as more of a problem to people who do not personally have a hearing loss.

More deaf parents were sure they did not want PND for deafness than hearing parents. This could be for two reasons: the first, because deaf people may not see having a deaf child as a problem and so may not have a need to find out the hearing status of the baby before it is born. The second, because the whole issue of genetic testing is seen to threaten the Deaf community, and showing an interest in this would contradict the generally negative feelings about the use of genetics (Jordan, 1991; Middleton, Hewison and Mueller, 1998). Researchers also report that people with a genetic condition are more likely to disagree with PND for that condition than those without the condition (Michie and Marteau, 1999).

The above figures imply that a genetic counselling service would mainly be catering for hearing patients or else those utilizing the medical model of deafness. There could be less of a demand from deaf patients, a percentage of whom could be culturally Deaf. Nevertheless it would still be important for the professionals involved with these families to have some training in deaf awareness, possibly with knowledge of BSL.

Not all patients who come for genetic counselling want PND. There are many other aspects to genetic counselling that deaf families would be interested in, such as information about the pattern of inheritance in their family and chances of having deaf or hearing children. Therefore, the potential demand from deaf and hearing families for genetic counselling could be higher in reality than the figures given above would suggest.

Reasons for having PND for deafness

The majority of all parents would have PND for deafness so they could prepare themselves for the child's needs or else prepare for the language (e.g. BSL) that the child could use. This could be seen as reassuring in that most would not wish to end the pregnancy if the test indicated the baby was likely to be deaf – a fear of members of the Deaf community (Middleton, Hewison and Mueller, 1998).

Since current PND techniques involve a risk of miscarriage, questions are raised about whether it would be appropriate for participants to be offered such testing if they are not intending to act on the information. It also suggests that participants may not have been aware that PND involved any risks to the pregnancy when they gave their answers.

Termination of pregnancy for hearing status

One deaf parent (1%) and 32 hearing parents (8%) said they would consider having a TOP if the fetus were found to be deaf. None of the parents would consider a TOP for 'hearingness'. Therefore, the potential uptake of PND for deafness with selective TOP for hearing status is low. For the one participant who was deaf, it is possible that they may have had such a negative experience of living with a hearing loss, perhaps growing up in isolation and experiencing discrimination, that they did not want to take the risk of passing on deafness to their children. For hearing participants, it is possible that their experience of living with deafness in the family was negative and so they too did not want to risk having more deaf children.

Interest in PND for deafness and preference for having deaf or hearing children

Parents who were interested in PND for deafness generally preferred to have hearing children. However, three (9%) deaf parents said they were interested in PND for deafness and also preferred to have deaf children. These participants were culturally Deaf. This means that there is a theoretical chance that some deaf people may use genetic technology to enable them to have deaf children. However, when asked specifically whether they would have a TOP if the fetus was found to be hearing, i.e. if they wanted to actively choose to have deaf children, all declined. In the larger study of results published elsewhere, three deaf participants (2% of sample) said they would consider TOP for 'hearingness' (i.e. they preferred to have deaf children) (Middleton, Hewison and Mueller, 2001; Middleton, 2004).

Ethical debate

A discussion about the ethical issues relating to general prenatal genetic testing is well established (e.g. American Medical Association, 1994; Burgess, 1994; Kapp, 1994; Macer, 1998). However, additional ethical dilemmas are posed by issues specifically pertinent to deafness, e.g. the intention of deaf parents to use genetic technology to allow them to have deaf children. This has been debated by Davis (1997) and is summarized here.

Most genetic counsellors are committed to the model of non-directive counselling, so facilitating patient autonomy. However, most genetic counsellors also tend to have certain beliefs about disability, e.g. that it is better to not have cystic fibrosis than to have it, or that it is better to be hearing than deaf. Therefore, when faced with an issue that turns preconceptions about disability around, such as with deaf parents wanting to use genetic technology to allow them to have deaf children and feeling that deafness is the norm and to hear is a disability, a conflict of morals and ethical beliefs arises. Does the parent's right to autonomy override the child's right to beneficence (good quality of life)? Who is to judge that deaf children born into a deaf family would be worse off than if they had been hearing? Davis argues that the conflict between autonomy and beneficence is insoluble, and that the real issue is between parental autonomy and the child's future autonomy. The debate does not need to concentrate on whether a deaf child born into a deaf family would be better off or not, but rather whether deliberately closing options for a child still leaves them with freedom of their choice (an 'open future'). Davis (1997) concluded:

> If deafness is considered a disability, one that substantially narrows a child's career, marriage, and cultural options in the future, then deliberately creating a deaf child counts as a moral harm. If Deafness is considered a culture, as Deaf activists would have us agree, then deliberately creating a Deaf child who will have only very limited options to move outside of that culture, also counts as a moral harm. A decision, made before a child is even born, that confines her forever to a narrow group of people and a limited choice of careers, so violates the child's right to an open future that no Genetic Counseling team should acquiesce in it. The very value of autonomy that grounds the ethics of Genetic Counseling should preclude assisting parents in a project that so dramatically narrows the autonomy of the child to be.

Choosing to have deaf children

Although ethicists may argue that using genetic technology to have deaf children is morally wrong, it does not stop deaf people preferring to have deaf children. A deaf lesbian couple in the USA wanted to increase their chance of having a deaf child by choosing to have artificial insemination from a male deaf friend; subsequently a deaf son was born, to their great delight (McLellan, 2002). This process used knowledge of genetic inheritance to create a situation that they wanted, although they did not actively have any genetic manipulation or intervention. This case caused international debate about the ethics of deliberately creating what to some people felt was a 'disabled' child. Some comments on the case were:

> Couples who select disabled rather than non-disabled offspring should be allowed to make those choices, even though they may be having a child with worse life prospects (Savulescu, 2002).

> Couples should not be allowed to select neither for nor against deafness (Anstey, 2002).

> Deaf people are behaving like hearing people. They feel good about themselves and want to have babies like them. Why should they be morally blamed? (Fletcher, 2002)

> To intentionally give a child a disability . . . is incredibly selfish (Ken Connor, president of the Family Research Council in Spriggs, 2002).

> Cultures are simply the kind of things to which we are born, and therefore to which the children of deaf parents, hearing or deaf, normally belong. Thus these parents are making a mistake in choosing deafness for their children. Given their own experience of isolation as children, however, it is a mistake which is understandable, and our reaction to them ought to be compassion, not condemnation (Levy, 2002).

There is currently no worldwide consensus of opinion on this issue.

Should termination of pregnancy for hearing status be illegal?

The majority of all participants from each group thought TOP for deafness or 'hearingness' should be illegal. Deaf participants were the most likely to think that TOP for deafness should be illegal.

Introducing the issue of legality gave participants the chance to demonstrate the strength of their feeling on TOP for hearing status. It is not suggested that the findings from this study should be used in a potential 'fight' to make TOP for hearing status illegal. The aim of the question was to offer an opportunity for participants to demonstrate their views. Some participants commented that they felt that making TOP illegal was too extreme, and said they would prefer to say that TOP for hearing status should not be made available. It is difficult to know how this would be policed and who should decide what tests would be available or not – the government, individual doctors, society?

Other research has introduced the issue of legality for TOP. Stern et al. (2002) asked deaf and hearing participants to say what they thought of TOP for deafness and 'hearingness' and whether this should be illegal. The responses fitted exactly the same pattern as found in the present study, with approximately 80% of deaf participants in both studies saying that TOP for a hearing fetus should be illegal when a deaf child is preferred and 72–85% thought TOP for deafness should be illegal.

If the attitudes shown in this study were a reflection of behaviour, then the potential impact of TOP for hearing status on health services would be small. This, together with the obvious strength of feeling against TOP for hearing status from most participants, questions whether or not this is a service that should be available. If TOP for hearing status were not allowed, then it is questionable whether PND should be made available if it is only to be used for the sake of information so that the parents can prepare themselves.

Termination of pregnancy for different scenarios

Looking at the overall attitudes of both deaf and hearing parents towards TOP for different scenarios, deafness was seen as a condition which is not as 'serious' as blindness, Huntington's Disease or Tay–Sachs disease but slightly more 'serious' than choosing to have a deaf baby or a baby of a specific sex. For hearing parents, deafness was more 'serious' than a treatable physical defect but, for deaf parents, it was less 'serious' than this.

The fact that deaf parents saw deafness as less 'serious' than the other given conditions is not surprising, since many studies have shown that people with a condition have different attitudes to those without the condition. For example, people with CF are less likely to consider TOP for CF than their parents. Therefore, they view CF as less 'serious' than do their parents (Conway, Allenby and Pond, 1994). Such differing attitudes highlight the difficulty that governments, doctors or society faces if asked to decide what conditions PND should be offered for. The fact that some individuals view the same scenarios differently supports the idea that it would be better to leave decisions regarding PND to the individual rather than encouraging genetics professionals or governments into deciding where the line should be drawn with regard to what *they* think is acceptable for PND.

Deaf parents of deaf children were less interested in TOP for deafness than hearing parents of deaf children, yet their interest in TOP for all the other conditions was approximately the same as for hearing parents of deaf children. This indicates that being deaf may not alter attitudes in general to TOP for conditions other than deafness itself. This point is important in the context of genetic counselling, since it means that no assumptions should be made about the opinions of 'disabled' people towards PND and selective TOP for conditions that they do not have; they may be just as interested in using PND as other 'non-disabled' people.

Where does PND change from being acceptable to not being acceptable? For example, it is acceptable for many people that PND is available for serious life-threatening conditions such as CF (Watson et al., 1992a), but it is not so clear what should happen with other conditions that are not life threatening. Research has shown that both the public and professionals (geneticists, obstetricians and ethicists) agreed with the use of PND with the offer of TOP for conditions involving significant degrees of intellectual and/or physical disability such as Down's syndrome, anencephaly or CF (Michie et al., 1995). However, there was very little support for PND for 'non-disease' characteristics such as homosexuality, low intelligence or two missing fingers (Michie et al., 1995). The dilemma occurs with conditions that are not easily defined as either 'serious' or 'non-serious'. To some people, deafness would be considered a condition where PND was appropriate, whereas to others it is not. For conditions where PND is possible, and a parent has a good argument for using it, it would usually be possible for them to have it if one follows the philosophy of non-directive genetic counselling. There are no government guidelines in the UK indicating those conditions for which PND and TOP should not be available.

Attitudes of geneticists and genetic counsellors

A large (n = 2903) international study of geneticists and genetic counsellors looked at the attitudes towards PND for many different scenarios including deafness (Wertz and Fletcher, 1998). Professionals were asked what they would do if they were approached by a deaf couple seeking PND in order to have a deaf child, with the intention of aborting a hearing fetus if the prenatal test showed this. Among the British genetics professionals, 9% would perform a prenatal test for this couple and 69% would refuse to do prenatal genetic testing for them. From an international perspective, the top four countries which would perform PND for the deaf couple included 38% of geneticists from Italy, 38% from Israel, 35% from the USA and 33% of those from Russia (Wertz and Fletcher, 1998). Those who said they would offer the testing argued from an 'autonomy' perspective, i.e. if the parents were able to make a fully informed, autonomous decision then the professionals felt they could not refuse them use of the technology (personal communication, Wertz and Fletcher, 1999)

Assessment of support

Deaf parents were more likely than hearing parents to feel they received support from family and friends at the time of diagnosis of deafness in their child. This could be because deaf parents were more likely to have deaf friends who understood the impact of the diagnosis. It may also mean that to many hearing parents, having a deaf child confers such shock and uncertainty, that more support is required than a deaf parent would need.

The results were less clear on attitudes towards receiving enough support from health professionals. Slightly more hearing parents than deaf parents said they did not receive enough support from health professionals, although this association was not significant. This could be because hearing parents actually needed more support than deaf parents because it was more of a shock to them to have their child diagnosed as deaf. If they needed more support, then they are less likely to feel that the support they did receive was sufficient. One hearing parent commented that health professionals were unhelpful because they saw deafness only in medical terms, rather than looking at the bigger picture, such as the impact on the family.

Impact of deafness on the child and family

Hearing parents were the most likely to think their deaf child was disadvantaged, whereas deaf parents were more likely to think that there were advantages and disadvantages to the deafness in their child. Deaf parents have personal experience of a hearing loss and so know more about how to cope with this. One hearing parent commented that the advantage of being deaf was that they could be part of the Deaf world, whereas because they were deaf they were disadvantaged in the hearing world.

A deaf parent commented that it was an advantage that their child was deaf because the rest of the family was deaf and so the child was not left out. However, several hearing parents commented that deafness was a disadvantage because of communication problems and feelings of isolation within hearing society.

With regard to the burden of deafness, deaf parents were the most likely to say that deafness caused no burden to them, whereas hearing parents were most likely to think the burden ranged from very little to very great. This implied that deaf parents cope better with the deafness in their child than hearing parents, which was to be expected. Schum (1991) reports that deaf children of deaf parents may be more likely to develop shared communication from birth and therefore less likely to encounter psychological problems associated with social interaction. However, deaf children of hearing parents are less likely to be as successful at this and so such parents are more likely to encounter problems with their child (Schum, 1991). Brand and Coetzer give details of a study by Hamner and Turner showing that attachment bonds between a child and their hearing mother may be weaker for deaf children than hearing children (Hamner and Turner, 1990, cited in Brand and Coetzer, 1994). This fits into the findings that hearing parents find the deafness more of a burden to deal with than deaf parents. (See also Chapter 5.)

Comments from parents showed a mixed response to the deafness in the child. One culturally Deaf parent said that having a deaf child was 'a joy' and therefore no burden whatsoever, while another deaf parent said they had the burden of stress and anxiety over education needs. A hearing parent said that trying to access the right education, speech therapy and learn a new language (BSL) was also a burden. Two hearing mothers said that the burden of deafness was so great on the family that their marriage had broken up and their husbands had left. This shows how in some instances deafness can be such a problem that it destroys a family. This finding is not new: Brand and Coetzer (1994) report that a shortfall in communication between the parent and deaf child often occurs and can put enormous stress on family relations.

Cure for deafness

Hearing parents were much more likely to want to have a cure for deafness for their child than deaf parents. This was to be expected since, as shown above, deafness seems more of a negative experience to hearing parents than to deaf parents. The comments given by the parents supported this result. One hearing parent said their child desperately wanted to be able to hear music and know what other children his age were saying. On the other hand, one culturally Deaf parent said that, by raising the issue of a cure or treatment for deafness, self-esteem in a deaf child would be damaged because they would feel that there is something wrong with them.

Experience of gaining a diagnosis and education

More deaf parents thought the experience of gaining a diagnosis of deafness in their child was easy or straightforward, whereas hearing parents were more likely to think the process was difficult or complicated. This implies that deaf parents may have had more of an awareness of the process of obtaining a diagnosis, and would probably have more knowledge of the medical system that the child would have to go through. For hearing parents, however, usually with no previous experience of ENT or audiology and little understanding of the different professionals who would have to be seen, the experience may be more daunting and difficult. There is also the chance that, because deaf parents have a hearing loss themselves, they are more likely to be taken seriously by the health professionals when they suggest that their child may be deaf. Hearing parents, with little or no knowledge of deafness, may be labelled as neurotic for repeatedly asking that their child be tested for deafness, especially if the child has already passed the health visitor's 'distraction test'.

The National Deaf Children's Society, in the UK reports that a late diagnosis is one of the issues that worries parents most (Watkin et al., 1995). Comments from parents in the current study showed that a late diagnosis caused much anxiety. One hearing parent said that they had to take their child to the hospital six times before the health professionals were convinced that the child was deaf. The result was that hearing aids were not given until the child was 3 years old. One hearing mother said she was ignored when she suggested that her child was deaf, and was told that she had postnatal depression. Eventually the child was diagnosed nearly 2 years later. These findings show that more attention should be paid by health professionals to the needs of parents at the time of diagnosis. Barringer et al. (1993) showed that 80% of successful diagnoses were initiated by parents seeking out a referral. This shows that the suspicions of parents need to be listened to at a time when deafness is suspected. More care should also be given to explaining not only the medical procedures and the medical impact of deafness but also the social and communicative impact; these issues could help improve service provision.

Factors affecting parents' interest in PND for deafness

Deaf parents who were interested in PND for deafness were more likely to prefer to have hearing children, see their deaf children as disadvantaged, feel an actual burden of having a child who is deaf and want a cure for deafness in their child.

The association found between the actual burden of deafness and an interest in PND for deafness for deaf parents is comparable to results of other work looking at the burden of disease. Denayer et al. (1992) showed an association between perceived burden of raising a child with CF and acceptance of TOP for CF; Meryash (1992) showed that women who perceived having a child with fragile X the most burdensome were more likely to consider TOP for it and Evers-Kiebooms et al. (1993) showed that the greater the perceived burden of bringing up a child with a physical or mental handicap the greater the interest in PND and TOP. Therefore, the results from the main study fit in with the published literature on other conditions.

Hearing parents interested in PND for deafness were more likely to see TOP for deafness as acceptable, find the communication with their child less than perfect (ranging from successful to poor) and find the experience of obtaining education for their child difficult or complicated. This finding is important since it shows that if more attention was paid to ensuring the process of obtaining education flowed more easily and was less stressful, then hearing parents may be less interested in having PND for deafness. This is of startling importance to education authorities and indicates that the service offered by such authorities needs to be reviewed.

Looking at all the results from parents collectively, it is possible to infer that many factors influence interest in PND for deafness. If such factors were changed then interest in PND for deafness might decline. For example, there may be less interest in PND for deafness if parents were better able to see their child as advantaged or less of a burden, or if they felt that communication with their child was easier or there were more straightforward processes to obtaining appropriate education. It should be possible for all professionals dealing with deaf families to look at these issues and improve the service they offer.

Implications for service provision

The process of obtaining a diagnosis and education for the deaf child can be stressful for parents and could be much improved with more care and support from professionals who deal with these processes. With more understanding of the parents' point of view, a better service can be offered. This could be achieved if professionals were made aware of parents' experiences either through specific incorporation of this subject in their training or by using techniques such as focus group discussion involving parents, for professionals currently practising.

There needs to be more input from health professionals to improve communication between parents and deaf children. This could contribute towards helping parents to see the deafness in their child as less of a burden or disadvantage to the child, and could help parents feel they are supported by their health professional. Support with communication could be done through the current services offered by teachers and social workers for the deaf. However, the services offered by such professionals vary, depending on geographical location. Communication issues could easily be addressed if input from teachers and social workers for the deaf were made more available, so allowing more time to be spent with each child. Charities and clubs for the deaf could take a more active role in supporting parents of deaf children. Diverting funds specifically to this cause could help with this.

Deaf awareness could be incorporated more into the training of professionals who see deaf families. This might involve learning about the different sorts of interpreters that are appropriate for deaf or hard-of-hearing individuals (e.g. BSL, SSE, lip-speaker, etc.), the dynamics of using an interpreter in a clinic session, the importance of using clear lip patterns in speech, the use of eye contact and an understanding of how the usual interactions with clients have to be altered to accommodate a hearing loss. In addition to all the practical considerations, it would be useful for professionals to have an awareness of behavioural and attitudinal differences of the culturally Deaf. Also, this would be in keeping with the demands of the British Deaf Association Policy Statement on Genetics (BDA, 2003).

A need for earlier diagnosis

If a test during pregnancy is not possible, then a test at birth could be considered the next best thing. Watkin et al. (1995) report that many parents of deaf children would have preferred the deafness to be diagnosed earlier rather than later, with many parents showing an interest in neonatal screening. Even if PND for deafness is not offered because of the ethical implications, there is a need for earlier diagnosis so that parents can prepare for their child's needs. The earlier the diagnosis the more time there is for the parents to come to terms with it and start preparing with how they are going to cope. This could be done by learning about language, e.g. by learning BSL, or learning how to teach speech to a mildly deaf child.

The end of deafness?

Many deaf people fear that genetics will be used to wipe out the Deaf community (Grundfast and Rosen, 1992; Middleton, Hewison and Mueller, 1998). This could only be a possibility if all deafness was due to genetic causes and everyone who was pregnant used PND with selective TOP for deaf fetuses, or used in vitro fertilization with preimplantation genetic diagnosis (PGD) to select only embryos without deafness-causing genes. Since deafness is due to environmental and genetic causes, and there are probably still many relevant genes that have yet to be discovered, it is likely there will be deafness in society for a long time to come. However, the results discussed in this chapter show that very few people from an at-risk population with knowledge of deafness would be interested in PND with selective TOP for deafness. Most deaf parents would not have PND and approximately half of hearing parents would. Of those who would have PND, only a very small minority would actually have a TOP for deafness. Therefore, the possibility that the Deaf community would be wiped out by PND and selective TOP of deaf fetuses is not supported by these results.

Actively choosing to abort a wanted pregnancy because it has the 'wrong' hearing status would be traumatic for any couple. It is possible that attitudes studied here are not good predictors of behaviour. When couples are actually faced with a pregnancy it is questionable whether they would, in reality, have a TOP because the baby has the 'wrong' hearing status. Nevertheless, these results demonstrate the strength of feeling on the subject. Given that PGD is detached both physically, and in time, from a pregnancy where a baby is alive and growing in the mother, it is possible that parents may choose to select on the basis of hearing status more readily than actually having a TOP. It would be useful for health professionals involved with PGD to have an awareness of the views of deaf families and their hearing relatives.

PGD has already been granted as acceptable for a hearing couple who want to avoid having deaf children. Such a couple, from Australia, were both carriers for faults in the connexin 26 gene and won the right to use PGD to ensure that any embryos with the deafness-causing genes were selected out (Australasian Bioethics Information, 2002; Kelly, 2002). The couple went ahead with this procedure but to date it is not thought that a successful pregnancy has been achieved (Noble, 2003).

Bioethicists have since declared that this policy to offer PGD for deafness is discriminatory and deafness is not a valid reason for such selection (Kelly, 2002). The Infertility Treatment Authority in Melbourne who granted permission for the use of this technology said it can be available to help hearing couples have hearing children but it would not be available to help Deaf couples wanting to have deaf children (ITA, 2003). This does appear to discriminate against potential Deaf couples who on the basis of their cultural heritage may prefer to have deaf children.

Should PND for deafness be available?

Genetics professionals find themselves in an impossible position if they subscribe to the model of non-directive counselling. If a Deaf person requests PND or PGD for hearing status with the intention of selecting for a deaf embryo/fetus, then a geneticist who is being truly non-directive and respecting client autonomy could enable them to do this. However, if genetics professionals are not comfortable offering services for indications such as deafness, the wrong sex or a treatable physical defect, then they will come under criticism for 'playing God' and denying some individuals access to services/options they feel strongly that they should have a right to use.

If individuals wish to use genetics services then they should only do so with adequate counselling to explore all the issues relating to the psychological consequences of their choices. If this is done, then any decisions regarding PND or PGD are carried out by fully informed individuals with complete autonomy. It is up to them to challenge the health professionals concerned if the services they wish to use are not readily available. If the current philosophy of non-directive genetic counselling is to be maintained, individuals must be allowed to make decisions that are right for them, giving them control of their own lives and allowing them to live with the consequences.

Conclusions

This chapter has documented the attitudes of deaf and hearing parents of deaf children towards the potential interest in using PND for deafness and opinion on TOP for hearing status. Although the focus of this chapter was to assess attitudes towards these issues, the results show that these findings must not be looked at in isolation. Although it is often of interest to clinicians and purchasers to know whether there is demand for a certain test, these figures are of no use unless they are looked at within the context of the bigger picture: understanding how deafness impacts on individuals and families. This is discussed further in Chapters 5–8.

The results have shown that interest in using PND was low. However, some participants said they would use PND for deafness and of these most would do so only to prepare themselves for their child. A minority had the intention of aborting a fetus if it was found to have a hearing status they did not want. Participants who were interested in PND for deafness tended to see deafness as a burden or disadvantage and struggled to communicate with the deaf children they already had. They were inclined to view living with deafness as a struggle, and something they did not want for future children. However, despite the negative picture created about deafness many participants also viewed deafness positively. Culturally Deaf participants were particularly optimistic about their situation and felt that being deaf was not a disability at all. This shows that deafness is not a condition that is clearly detrimental. It is therefore possible that with extra support and funding to help the parents of newly diagnosed deaf children a better image of deafness could be created.

It is vital to learn about the diversity of attitudes that different people affected by deafness have, so that appropriate and effective services can be developed within the many agencies involved with deaf individuals and their families. This work contributes evidence, which can be used as a basis for improving services for deaf people.

References

American Medical Association (1994) Ethical issues related to prenatal genetic testing. Archives of Family Medicine 3: 633–642.

Anstey KW (2002) Are attempts to have impaired children justifiable? Journal of Medical Ethics 28: 286–288.

Arnos KS, Israel J, Cunningham M (1991) Genetic counselling for the deaf: medical and cultural considerations. Annals of the New York Academy of Sciences 630: 212–222.

Arnos KS, Israel J, Devlin L, Wilson MP (1992) Genetic counselling for the deaf. Otolaryngologic Clinics of North America 25: 953–971.

Atkins DV (1994) Counseling children with hearing loss and their families. In: Clark JG, Martin FN (eds) Effective Counseling in Audiology. Perspectives and practice. Prentice Hall, Englewood Cliffs, NJ, pp. 116–146.

Australasian Bioethics Information (2002) Designer babies/go ahead to screen out deafness. Australasian Bioethics Information Newsletter, 27 September.

Bahan B (1989) What if . . . Alexander Graham Bell had gotten his way? In: Wilcox S (ed.) American Deaf Culture. Linstock Press, Silver Spring, MD, pp. 83–87.

Barringer DG, Strong CJ, Blair JC, Clark TC, Watkins S (1993) Screening procedures used to identify children with hearing loss. American Annals of the Deaf 138: 420–426.

BDA (2003) Policy Statement on Genetics. Departmental publication. British Deaf Association, London.

Brand HJ, Coetzer MA (1994) Parental response to their child's hearing impairment. Psychological Reports 75: 1363–1368.

Brunger JW, Murray GS, O'Riordan M et al. (2000) Parental attitudes toward genetic testing for pediatric deafness. American Journal of Human Genetics 67: 1621–1625.

Burgess MM (1994) Ethical issues in prenatal testing. Clinical Biochemistry 27(2): 87–91.

CADS (1987) Annual Survey of Hearing Impaired Children and Youths. Gallaudet University, Washington, DC.

Chapple A, May C, Campion P (1995) Lay understanding of genetic disease: a British study of families attending a genetic counseling service. Journal of Genetic Counseling 4: 281–301.

Christiansen JB (1991) Sociological implications of hearing loss. Annals of the New York Academy of Sciences 630: 230–235.

Chung CS, Brown KS (1970) Family studies of early childhood deafness ascertained through the Clarke School for the deaf. American Journal of Human Genetics 22: 357–366.

Cohen MM, Gorlin RJ (1995) Epidemiology, aetiology and genetic patterns. In: Gorlin RJ, Toriello HV, Cohen MM (eds) Hereditary Hearing Loss and its Syndromes. Oxford University Press, Oxford, pp. 9-21.

Conway SP, Allenby K, Pond MN (1994) Patient and parental attitudes toward genetic screening and its implications at an adult CF centre. Clinical Genetics 45: 308-312.

Dagan O, Hichner H, Levi H et al. (2002) Genetic testing for hearing loss: different motivations for the same outcome. American Journal of Medical Genetics 113: 137-143.

Das VK (1996) Aetiology of bilateral sensorineural hearing impairment in children: a 10 year study. Archives of Disease in Childhood 74: 8-12.

Davis DS (1997) Genetic dilemmas and the child's right to an open future. Hastings Central Report 27(2): 7-15.

Denayer L, Evers-Kiebooms G, Boeck K De, Berghe H Van den (1992) Reproductive decision making of aunts and uncles of a child with CF: genetic risk perception and attitudes toward carrier identification and prenatal diagnosis. American Journal of Medical Genetics 44: 104-111.

Denoyelle F, Marlin S et al. (1999) Clinical features of the prevalent form of childhood deafness, DFNB1, due to a connexin-26 defect: implications for genetic counselling. Lancet 353: 1298-1303.

Denoyelle F, Weil D, Maw MA et al. (1997) Prelingual deafness: high prevalence of a 30delG mutation in the connexin 26 gene. Human Molecular Genetics 6: 2173-2177.

Dolnick E (1993) Deafness as culture. Atlantic Monthly 272(3): 37-53.

Estivill X, Fortina P et al. (1998) Connexin-26 mutations in sporadic and inherited sensorineural deafness. Lancet 351: 394-398.

Evers-Kiebooms G, Denayer L et al. (1993) Community attitudes towards prenatal testing for congenital handicap. Journal of Reproductive and Infant Psychology 11: 21-30.

Fletcher JC (2002) Deaf like us: the Duchesneau-McCullough case. L'Observatoire de la genetique – Cadrages 5 (July/August).

Fraser GR (1964) A study of causes of deafness amongst 2355 children in special schools. In: Fisch L (ed.) Research in Deafness in Children. Blackwell Science, Oxford, pp. 10-13.

Fraser GR (1976) The causes of profound deafness in childhood. Johns Hopkins University Press, Baltimore, MD.

Gibson WPR (1991) Opposition from deaf groups to the cochlear implant. Medical Journal of Australia 155: 212-214.

Green JM (1992) Principles and practicalities of carrier screening: attitudes of recent parents. Journal of Medical Genetics 29: 313-319.

Grundfast KM, Rosen J (1992) Ethical and cultural considerations in research on hereditary deafness. Otolaryngologic Clinics of North America 25: 973-978.

Harper PS (1993) Practical Genetic Counselling. Butterworth-Heinemann, Oxford.

Israel J (ed.) (1995) An Introduction to Deafness: a manual for genetic counsellors. Genetic Services Centre, Gallaudet University, Washington, DC.

ITA (2003) Policy in relation to the use of preimplantation genetic diagnosis for genetic testing. Departmental Policy. Infertility Treatment Authority, Melbourne, Victoria, Australia: Ita@ita.org.au.

Johnson RE, Erting CJ (1989) Ethnicity and socialization in a classroom for deaf children. In: Lucas C (ed.) The Sociolinguistics of the Deaf Community. Academic Press, San Diego, CA, pp. 41-83.

Jordan IK (1991) Ethical issues in the genetic study of deafness. Annals of the New York Academy of Sciences 630: 236–239.

Kaback M, Zippin D, Boyd P, Cantor R (1984) Attitudes Toward Prenatal Diagnosis of CF Among Parents of Affected Children. John Wiley, New York.

Kapp MB (1994) Ethical and legal implications of advances in genetic testing technology. Legal Medicine 305–319.

Kelley PM, Harris DJ, Comer BC et al. (1998) Novel mutations in the connexin 26 gene (GJB2) that cause autosomal recessive (DFNB1) hearing loss. American Journal of Human Genetics 62: 792–799.

Kelly J (2002) Designer baby to have perfect hearing. Herald Sun (Melbourne), 21 September.

Kessler S (1997) Psychological aspects of genetic counselling, XI. Nondirectiveness revisited. American Journal of Medical Genetics 72: 164–171.

Kluwin TN, Gaustad MG (1991) Predicting family communication choices. American Annals of the Deaf 136(1): 28–34.

Koester LS, Meadow-Orlans KP (1990) Parenting a deaf child: stress, strength, and support. In: Moores D, Meadow-Orlans KP (eds) Educational and Developmental Aspects of Deafness. Gallaudet University Press, Washington, DC, pp. 299–320.

Lane H (1984) When the Mind Hears: a history of the deaf. Random House, New York.

Lench N, Houseman M, Newton V, Van Camp G, Mueller R (1998) Connexin-26 mutations in sporadic non-syndromal sensorineural deafness [letter]. Lancet 351: 415.

Levy N (2002) Deafness, culture and choice. Journal of Medical Ethics 28: 284–285.

Luterman DM, Ross M (1991) When Your Child is Deaf. A guide for parents. York, Parkton, MD.

Macer DRJ (1998) Ethics and prenatal diagnosis. In: Milunsky A (ed.) Genetic Disorders and the Fetus: diagnosis, prevention and treatment. Johns Hopkins University Press, Baltimore, MD, pp. 999–1024.

McLellan F (2002) Controversy over deliberate conception of deaf child. Lancet 359: 1315.

Marazita M, Ploughman L, Rawlings B et al. (1993) Genetic epidemiological studies of early-onset deafness in the US school-age population. American Journal of Medical Genetics 46: 486–491.

Marteau T, Richards M (eds) (1996) The Troubled Helix: social and psychological implications of the new human genetics. Cambridge University Press, Cambridge.

Martinez A, Linden J, Schimmenti LA, Palmer CGS (2003) Attitudes of the broader hearing, deaf and hard of hearing community toward genetic testing for deafness. Genetics in Medicine 5: 106–112.

Meadow KP (1976) Personality and social development of deaf persons. In: Bolton B (ed.) Psychology of deafness for rehabilitation counselors. University Park Press, Baltimore, MD, pp. 67–80.

Meadow-Orlans KP (1990) Research on developmental aspects of deafness. In: Moores D, Meadow-Orlans KP (eds) Educational and Developmental Aspects of Deafness. Gallaudet University Press, Washington, DC, pp. 283–298.

Meryash DL (1992) Characteristics of fragile X relatives with different attitudes toward terminating an affected pregnancy. American Journal of Mental Retardation 96: 528–535.

Michie S, Drake H, Bobrow M, Marteau T (1995) A comparison of public and professionals' attitudes towards genetic developments. Public Understanding of Science 4: 243–253.

Michie S, Marteau TM (1999) The choice to have a disabled child. American Journal of Human Genetics 65: 1204–1207.

Middleton A (1999) Attitudes of deaf and hearing individuals towards issues surrounding genetic testing for deafness. PhD Thesis, Leeds University, UK.

Middleton A (2004) Deaf and hearing adults' attitudes towards genetic testing for deafness. In: Van Cleve JV (ed.) Genetics, Disability and Deafness. Washington, DC: Gallaudet University Press, pp. 127–147.

Middleton A, Hewison J, Mueller R (1998) Attitudes of deaf adults toward genetic testing for hereditary deafness. American Journal of Human Genetics 63: 1175–1180.

Middleton A, Hewison J, Mueller RF (2001) Pre-natal genetic testing for inherited deafness – what is the potential demand? Journal of Genetic Counseling 10(2): 121–131.

Mindel ED, Feldman V (1987) The impact of deaf children on their families. In: Mindel ED, Vernon M (eds) They Grow in Silence: understanding deaf children and adults. Pro-Ed, Austin, TX.

Mohay H (1991) Deafness in children [letter]. Medical Journal of Australia 155: 59.

Newton VE (1985) Aetiology of bilateral sensorineural hearing loss in young children. Journal of Laryngology and Otology 10(Suppl): 1–57.

Noble T (2003) Embryos screened for deafness – a quiet first for Australia. Sydney Morning Herald, 11 July.

Padden C (1980) The Deaf Community and the Culture of Deaf People. In: Wilcox S (ed.) American Deaf Culture. Linstock Press, Silver Spring, MD, pp. 1–16.

Parving A (1984) Aetiologic diagnosis in hearing-impaired children – clinical value and application of a modern programme. International Journal of Pediatric Otorhinolaryngology 7: 29–38.

Prezant TR, Agapian JV, Bohlman MC et al. (1993) Mitochondrial ribosomal RNA mutation associated with antibiotic-induced and non-syndromic deafness. Nature Genetics 4: 289–294.

Reardon W (1998) Connexin 26 gene mutation and autosomal recessive deafness. Lancet 351: 383–384.

Richards M (1997) It runs in the family: lay knowledge about inheritance. In: Clarke A, Parsons E (eds) Culture, Kinship and Genes: towards cross-cultural genetics. Macmillan, Basingstoke, pp. 175–197.

Sacks O (1990) Seeing Voices: a journey into the world of the deaf. Harper Perennial, New York.

Sagi M, Shiloh S, Cohen T (1992) Application of the Health Belief Model in a study on parent's intentions to utilize prenatal diagnosis of cleft lip and or palate. American Journal of Medical Genetics 44: 326–333.

Savulescu J (2002) Deaf lesbians, 'designer disability', and the future of medicine. BMJ 325: 771–773.

Schein JD (1989) Family life. In: At Home among Strangers. Gallaudet University Press, Washington, DC, pp. 106–134.

Schroedel JG, Schiff W (1972) Attitudes towards deafness among several deaf and hearing populations. Rehabilitation Psychology 19(2): 59–70.

Schum RL (1991) Communication and social growth: a developmental model of social behavior in deaf children. Ear and Hearing 12: 320–327.

Sloman L, Springer S et al. (1993) Disordered communication and grieving in deaf member families. Family Process 32: 171–183.

Spriggs M (2002) Lesbian couple create a child who is deaf like them. Journal of Medical Ethics 28: 283.

Stephens D (1996) Audiological terms. European Workgroup on Genetics of Hearing Impairment Infoletter 2: 8–9.

Stern SJ, Arnos KS, Murrelle L et al. (2002) Attitudes of deaf and hard of hearing subjects towards genetic testing and prenatal diagnosis of hearing loss. Journal of Medical Genetics 39: 449–453.

Vernon M, Andrews J (1990) Psychodynamics surrounding the diagnosis of deafness. In: Vernon M, Andrews J (eds) Psychology of Deafness – understanding deaf and hard of hearing people. Longman, New York, pp. 119–136.

Watkin PM, Beckman A, Baldwin N (1995) The views of parents of hearing impaired children on the need for neonatal hearing screening. British Journal of Audiology 29: 259–262.

Watson EK, Mayall ES, Lamb J, Chapple J, Williamson R (1992a) Psychological and social consequences of community carrier screening programme for CF. Lancet 340: 217–220.

Watson EK, Marchant J, Bush A, Williamson B (1992b) Attitudes towards prenatal diagnosis and carrier screening for CF among the parents of patients in a paediatric CF clinic. Journal of Medical Genetics 29: 490–491.

Wertz DC, Fletcher JC (1998) Ethical and social issues in prenatal sex selection: a survey of geneticists in 37 nations. Social Science and Medicine 46: 255–273.

Wertz DC, Rosenfield JM, James SR, Erbe RW (1991) Attitudes toward abortion among parents of children with CF. American Journal of Public Health 81: 992–996.

Wheeler J (1998) The end of all hearing loss is in reach. Editorial. American Journal of Otology 19: 1–3.

CHAPTER 3

The International Classification of Functioning, Disability and Health as a conceptual framework for the impact of genetic hearing impairment

DAFYDD STEPHENS AND BERTH DANERMARK

The first serious attempt to provide a universal framework for consideration of the impact of disease or congenital anomalies of the individual came with the work of Philip Wood (e.g. Wood and Badley, 1978). This led to the development of a uniform terminology which was widely disseminated through the World Health Organization's *International Classification of Impairments, Disabilities and Handicaps* – ICIDH (WHO, 1980). Through the adoption of this framework, individuals working in different fields and in different countries were able to communicate using the same definitions and concepts. It represented a major advance in the area of the impact of health conditions on the individual's life.

The basic structure of the ICIDH is shown in Figure 3.1, which indicates a left-to-right progression by which an underlying health or inherited condition could result in an *abnormality or abnormalities* of structure or function. These in turn result in a *disability*, basically the impact of the disorder on what the patient is able to do in that domain (e.g. the hearing difficulties consequential on the hearing impairment). Thus a loss of basal turn outer hair cells is associated with a high-frequency hearing impairment and, from the individual's point of view, this gives him or her difficulties in hearing in the presence of background noise.

Such disabilities may then impact on a person's life, resulting in one or more *handicaps*. Again, taking the same example, difficulty hearing in

54

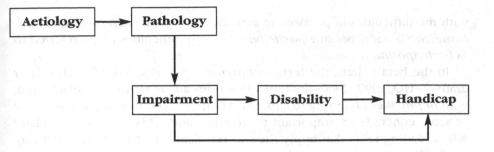

Figure 3.1. The relationship between the different components of the ICIDH (WHO, 1980).

background noise may result in the individual withdrawing from social activities, leading to social isolation, loneliness and depression. Handicap is thus the consequence of the condition on the individual's life.

The ICIDH also provided for a direct progression from *impairment* to *handicap*, bypassing *disability*. An example of this may be the fact that a spouse or partner always responds to the doorbell or telephone, without the person with hearing impairment realizing that this is happening. Consequently, when the partner is not around, the individual fails to hear friends trying to make contact, so eventually they give up the effort, and then they feel isolated without understanding why.

In addition, within the ICIDH, the term 'disablements' was used to refer to impairments, disabilities and handicaps collectively.

While the ICIDH was a major step forward (e.g. Stephens and Hétu, 1991), it had a number of weaknesses within the field of hearing impairment which were highlighted by those authors and others. These included the concept of secondary handicaps and the presence of feedback loops to take into account the impact of interventions and changes in circumstance. These were subsequently incorporated into a number of proposed developments of the ICIDH (e.g. Stephens and Kerr, 1995).

Another, more general, shortcoming was that – despite the fact that the model formally highlighted the interaction between an individual and his or her environment – the arrows in the figure indicated causal links and hence downplayed the environmental aspects of handicap.

These and other limitations consequently led to the development and publication, in 1997, of the Beta-1 draft of ICIDH-2 (WHO, 1997), which incorporated three important new concepts. The first of these was the use of a positive terminology outlining what the individual can do and does do, rather than what they cannot do. Thus, broadly, *disability* became *activity*, with the difficulties in performing activities defined as *activity limitations*. *Handicap* broadly became *participation*, with difficulties being referred to as *participation restrictions*.

In the Beta-1 draft, the term *impairment* was maintained, but in later drafts (WHO, 1999, 2000) the terms *functions* and *structures* were adopted, with *impairment* referring to anomalies of these. These changes in meaning of some concepts are important to bear in mind. This applies particularly when reading texts that apply the former meaning of *disability* (*activity limitations*) compared with newer texts, and particularly the final *International Classification of Functioning, Disability and Health* (ICF – WHO, 2001b), where *disability* is the umbrella term for *activity limitations* and *participation restrictions*.

The second major advance was the introduction of *contextual factors* – *environmental factors* (outside the person) and *personal factors* (within the person) – which could influence the levels of activities and participations as well as the interactions between them. These are dynamic influences, which can change at different times. The environmental contextual factors included inanimate (light and sound) and animate (significant others) components of the world around the individual, as well as the attitudes and structures of the society within which they live.

The third major improvement was the fact that changes and influences could occur in either direction, rather than the simple right-to-left progression found in the ICIDH. This enables, for example, the individual's activities both to influence their participations and to be influenced by them according to changing circumstances. Thus it takes into account both deteriorations in the individual's condition and the results of positive therapeutic or rehabilitative interventions. It also downplays the influence of the medical model which focused on aetiology, pathology and disease as the main causes and instead highlighted environmental factors, hence aiming at an integration of the medical and social models (WHO, 2001a, p. 20). This bridging of the gap between the medical and social models of disability and health has been welcomed by representatives of deaf people (e.g. Andersson, 2002).

ICIDH-2 went through a number of changes with the Beta-2 draft (1999), the pre-final draft (WHO, 2000) and the final draft (WHO, 2001a) released before the definitive version, in which it was renamed ICF, was published in the latter part of 2001 (WHO, 2001b). This final version is shown in Figure 3.2.

One overall weakness of this is the lack of an appropriate component summarizing the impact on the individual. From the neuro-rehabilitative standpoint, Wade (2003) has recently introduced the concept of *wellbeing*, bringing together the impact of impairments, activity limitations and partici-pation restrictions on the individual. However, Griggs (1998) has highlighted the dangers of applying the same concept of wellness to Deaf people.

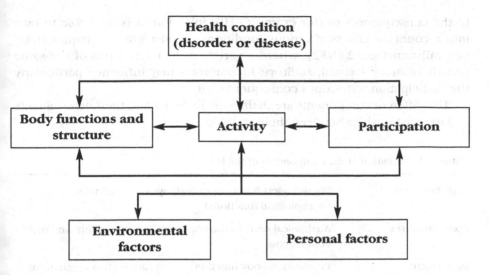

Figure 3.2. The ICF: final version.

Another weakness, highlighted by Nordenfelt (1997), among others, is the absence of a subjective dimension of functioning and disability (see also Ueda and Okawa, 2003).

Various attempts to appraise the system from an audiological or deaf blind context were affected by the changes between each new version of the development of ICF, which had a significant effect on its detailed application to this field (Stephens, 2001, 2002). However, several analyses relating to the final version of the ICF have been published (Stephens and Kerr, 2000; Patterson, 2001; Möller, 2003), and will be considered later where relevant. In particular, Patterson (2001) indicated how the ICF could be used to highlight the problems individual patients experienced using a framework/questionnaire based on the ICIDH-2/ICF. However, there is a potential for error when the problem-seeking is based on semions (symptoms evoked by direct questioning) as opposed to encouraging the patient to articulate their real problems. The latter approach has been adopted in the incorporation of the ICF into rehabilitation models by Stephens (2002) and by Kiessling et al. (2003) in audiological enablement (rehabilitation) and by Wade (2003) in neuro-rehabilitation.

The International Classification of Functioning, Disability and Health (ICF)

The overall structure of this classification is shown in Figure 3.2, which was designed to be as relevant to the effects of age-related hearing impairment as to the consequences of (for example) HIV infection. It is thus able to take into account the effects of various conditions as considered in Chapter 10 on neurofibromatosis 2 (NF2), where a variety of manifestations of the same genetic disorder – visual, auditory, locomotor – may influence particularly the participation restrictions consequent on it.

The different components are defined in Table 3.1 and their determinants and the relationships between them in Table 3.2.

Table 3.1. Definition of the components of the ICF

Body functions	Physiological functions of body systems (including psychological functions)
Body structures	Anatomical parts of the body such as organs, limbs and their components
Impairments	Problems in body function or structure such as a significant deviation or loss
Activity	The execution of a task or action by an individual
Activity limitations	Difficulties an individual may have in executing activities
Participation	Involvement in a life situation
Participation restrictions	Problems an individual may experience in involvement in life situations
Environmental factors	Make up the physical, social and attitudinal environment in which people live and conduct their lives
Personal factors	The particular background of an individual's life and living; they are composed of features of the individual that are not part of a health condition or health states

For most individuals considered in this book, the progression from disease and disorder to activities and participation will pass via the effect on structures or functions. However, for someone with a late-onset genetic disorder, particularly a severe and lethal condition such as NF2, just knowing that they have the mutated gene that causes the condition can have a major psychosocial impact on them. In this case, at a pre-symptomatic stage, disclosure of the genetic information, will affect the individual's participation as well as having an impact on aspects of their personal contextual factors.

For most patients who come within the scope of this book, however, it may be assumed that the psychosocial effects of the genetic disorder are a consequence of the impaired structure and function that it causes. Furthermore, most conditions under consideration have an impact principally on function,

Table 3.2. Determinants and relationships between the different components of the ICF

	Part 1: Functioning and disability		Part 2: Contextual factors	
	Body functions and structures	Activities and participation	Environmental factors	Personal factors
Components	Body functions and structures	Activities and participation	Environmental factors	Personal factors
Domains	Body functions Body structures	Life areas (tasks, actions)	External influences on functioning and disability	Internal influences on functioning and disability
Constructs	Change in body functions (physiological) / Change in body structures (anatomical)	Capacity — Executing tasks in a standard environment / Performance — Executing tasks in the current environment	Facilitating or hindering impact of features of the physical, social and attitudinal world	Impact of attributes of the person
Positive aspect	Functional and structural integrity	Activities Participation	Facilitators	Not applicable
	Functioning			
Negative aspect	Impairment	Activity limitation Participation restriction	Barriers/hindrances	Not applicable
	Disability			

the structural changes being at a microscopic level; so, for simplicity, we shall consider the conditions under the heading of impairments of function.

The broad headings relevant in the present context are shown in bold in Table 3.3. According to the ICF, many of the psychosocial factors that are discussed in the different chapters could be interpreted as being located in body functions (e.g. b152 on emotions). However, in our interpretation of the ICF, we locate these factors among personal contextual factors.

Table 3.3. Bodily functions

b1	Mental functions
b2	**Sensory functions and pain**
b3	Voice and speech functions
b4	Functions of the cardiovascular, haematological, immunological and respiratory systems
b5	Functions of the digestive, metabolic and endocrine systems
b6	Genitourinary and reproductive functions
b7	**Neuromusculoskeletal and movement-related functions**
b8	Functions of the skin and related structures

With the exclusion of these 'mental functions', the main areas of direct relevance are located in 'relevant sensory functions and pain', which are shown in Table 3.4.

Table 3.4. Relevant sensory functions and pain

Seeing and related functions:
     b210 Seeing functions
     b220 Sensations associated with the eye and adjoining structures

Hearing and vestibular functions:
     b230 Hearing functions
     b235 Vestibular functions
     b240 Sensations associated with hearing and vestibular function

b250–279 Additional sensory functions
b280 Pain

The two main areas in this context, in addition to aspects of hearing functions, which are relevant to all sections of the book, are hearing and vestibular functions (b230-249) and aspect of seeing function (b210-229) which are relevant to the chapters on deafblindness and NF2. NF2 can also have an impact on neuroskeletal and movement-related functions (b7).

Hearing and vestibular functions are shown in more detail in Table 3.5, to which phonophobia/hyperacusis is added as it otherwise disappeared in the course of the development of the ICF.

Table 3.5. Hearing and vestibular functions

b240	Sensations associated with hearing and vestibular function
	b2400 Ringing in ears or tinnitus
	b2404 Irritation in the ear
	b2405 Aural pressure
	ADD Phonophobia/hyperacusis

Disorders of both hearing and vision can have an impact on functions of equilibrium (b235), the former via balance disorders affecting the inner ear or vestibulocochlear nerve associated with the inner-ear lesions. Bilateral balance lesions are more likely to affect the individual when visual and proprioceptive inputs are restricted, such as in swimming, walking in the dark or walking over irregular surfaces. In the same way visual lesions, reducing this ability to compensate for vestibular dysfunction, can enhance balance abnormalities.

In addition, the heading 'sensations associated with hearing and vestibular function' (b240) includes tinnitus, which can have a major influence on the individual's life in certain cases. In particular, the psychological impact of the tinnitus, causing or enhancing underlying anxiety or depression, can interact with the individual's problems arising from their hearing or balance impairment.

Activities and participation

Within the ICF, the collective term for both activities and participations (as well as impairments) reverted to the rather confusing term *disabilities*. These are shown in Table 3.6.

Table 3.6. Activities and participation

d1	Learning and applying knowledge
d2	General tasks and demands
d3	Communication
d4	Mobility
d5	Self-care
d6	Domestic life
d7	Interpersonal interactions and relationships
d8	Major life areas
d9	Community, social and civic life

These may be considered in two ways. The main approach adopted in the ICF is to define *activity* as what the individual *can* do and *participation* as what they *do* do.

However, various alternatives to this are outlined in Annex 3 of the ICF (WHO, 2001b, pp. 234–237). In particular, for the purposes of the present study, the approach outlined as alternative 1 is perhaps the most relevant. In this the 'sets of Activity categories and Participation categories are determined by the user'. In the example presented, d1–4 (learning and applying knowledge; general tasks and demands; communication; and mobility) are categorized as activities and d5–9 (self-care; domestic life; interpersonal interactions; major life areas; and community, social and civic life) are classified as participations.

From a psychosocial context and in terms of reviewing the published literature, such an approach facilitates the process of analysis, with the domains of participation covering many of the psychosocial elements. These are illustrated in Table 3.7, in which self-care is of little relevance to the present discussion, except possibly in some cases of deafblindness and NF2. The key areas here are those of interpersonal interactions and relationships (d7), education, work and employment (d8), and various aspects of community, social and civic life (d9). In the last, the components of community life (d910) and leisure (d920), as well as religion and spirituality (d930), may be regarded as the most important.

Table 3.7. Relevant areas of participation

d5 Self-care

d6 Domestic life
    d610 Acquisition of necessities
    d630 Household tasks
    d650 Caring for household objects and assisting others

d7 Interpersonal interactions and relationships
    d710 General interpersonal relationships
    d730 Particular interpersonal relationships

d8 Major life areas
    d810 Education
    d840 Work and employment
    d860 Economic life

d9 Community, social and civic life
    d910 Community life
    d920 Recreation and leisure
    d930 Religion and spirituality
    d940 Human rights
    d950 Political life and citizenship

These are shown in more detail in Table 3.7. It is interesting to note that d730, 'particular interpersonal relationships', covers a wide range of relationships from strangers (d730) through to intimate relationships (d770), which includes romantic relationships (d7700), spousal relationships (d7701) and sexual relationships (d7702).

Contextual factors

Contextual factors are generally regarded as factors that influence the individual under consideration, but the ICF makes it clear that they may also be affected by the impact of the individual's condition.

Environmental contextual factors

In this respect, the element of environmental factors that will be particularly important is that of significant others who are closely involved with the individual on a daily basis (e3) and also their attitudes towards the affected individual and their condition (e4).

Here, as elsewhere in the context of contextual factors, there will be a two-way interaction. Thus the patient's problems will impact in some way on those around them, while in turn the attitude and approach of those around them will affect the impact of hearing loss on the patient. The classification of environmental factors shown in Table 3.8 highlights these areas, as well as the other relevant components. Within this, it may be seen that there are a range of factors – physical, human and institutional – which can influence the individual's reactions to hearing impairment. It is important not to ignore

Table 3.8. Relevant environmental factors

e1 Products and technology
    e115 Products and technology for personal use in daily living
    e125 Products and technology for communication

e2 Natural environment and human-made changes to environment
    e250 Sound

e3 Support and relationships

e4 Attitudes
    e410 Individual attitudes
    e460 Societal attitudes
    e465 Social norms, practices and ideologies

e5 Services, systems and policies
    e535 Communication services, systems and policies
    e575 General social support services, systems and policies
    e580 Health services, systems and policies

institutional provisions (e.g. free healthcare provision) which may have a significant impact on the help-seeking behaviour of the individual.

Table 3.9 highlights the different key groups of individuals who interact with a person with hearing impairment and who can affect and/or be affected by the impact of the individual's impairment.

Table 3.9. Support and relationships

e310	Immediate family
e315	Extended family
e320	Friends
e325	Acquaintances, peers, colleagues, neighbours and community members
e340	Personal care providers and personal assistants
e345	Strangers
e355	Health professionals
e360	Health-related professionals

Personal contextual factors

The question of the psychological impact of the various disorders is not clearly addressed within the ICF. We would argue that, in the same way as the individual's genetic hearing impairment may impact on those around them by an effect on environmental contextual factors, it can affect the individual *per se* in personal contextual factors. These have not, however, been categorized within the ICF. Stephens (2002) has attempted to address this with the classification shown in Table 3.10, based on a short paragraph on personal factors in the ICF (WHO, 2001b, p. 17).

Table 3.10. Personal contextual factors

Gender, race, age	Social background
Other health conditions	Education
Fitness	Profession
Lifestyle	Past and current experience
Habits	Overall behaviour pattern and character style
Upbringing	Individual psychological assets
Coping styles	

Within this outline, the psychosocial impact comes primarily in the areas of coping styles, overall behavioural pattern and individual psychological assets. Certainly this is reflected in the responses to a questionnaire asking individuals to list the effects of hearing impairment on their lives completed by elderly people with hearing impairment.

However, as with environmental factors, there is a two-way interaction. Thus, for example, inappropriate coping by the individual may result in their hearing impairment having a greater impact on them, leading to a loss of confidence, which should be considered under the heading 'Individual psychological assets'.

Overview

In this brief presentation a number of points have been overlooked in discussion to date, in addition to Wade's discussion of 'wellness'. Indeed, even within that context, Griggs (1998) has argued that deaf people's concept of wellness differs significantly from that of hearing people, particularly in relation to psychological wellness.

This leads to the question of whether individuals who have never experienced normal hearing (the congenitally deaf) can experience a handicap arising from it. In this respect it is of note (see Chapter 8) that individuals with Usher type 1 syndrome – profound congenital hearing impairment and progressive visual impairment – report the visual impairment and its consequences as the main problem. On the other hand, those with Usher type 2 syndrome – moderate hearing impairment and progressive visual impairment – report the hearing impairment as their major problem.

Using the ICF as our conceptual framework also has other consequences; one relates to the vocabulary. When reporting studies we use the vocabulary used by the author(s). However, when we comment on and discuss the findings, we try to use a language that is in harmony with the approach of the ICF, which aims to integrate the medical and social models, including the effort to use universalist terms. A second conceptual consequence is that it is unclear how to label people with hearing impairment according to their level of hearing. Our interpretation of the ICF is that, when talking about limitations in 'body functions' (i.e. physiological functions of body systems), we use concepts describing different levels of function. For instance, under 'hearing functions' (b230) seven different functions are described, e.g. sound detection (b2300), sound discrimination (b2301). These functions are rated from 0 (full functioning) to 4 (total absence of functioning) (Table 3.11). This means that, according to the ICF, it is relevant to talk about the level of hearing functions.

On the labelling issue, the WHO is also very clear that people have the right to be called what they choose (see WHO, 2001b, Annex 5, p. 242). The WHO is neutral regarding what people with hearing impairment call themselves. This means that a person scoring 0 on b2300–2309 might call herself Deaf. People who wish to indicate that they are culturally Deaf and belong to the Deaf community may therefore call themselves Deaf without any reference to the degree of hearing function.

Table 3.11. Quantitative aspects of the ICF applied to body function

Body function (e.g. speech discrimination b2304)	Degree
No impairment (none, absent, negligible)	0
Mild (slight, low)	1
Moderate (medium, fair)	2
Severe (high, extreme)	3
Complete (total)	4

However, ICF does not provide us with any guidelines describing the hearing function at a less detailed level (e.g. b230). In the scientific community there is a need for more summarizing concepts, and many different suggestions have appeared in audiological publications (e.g. Davis, 1970). Given the new ICF conceptual framework, these former descriptions are not always accurate. Moreover, no new conceptualization based on the ICF has so far appeared. However, it is beyond the scope of this book to solve this issue. Here we can indicate only the absence of descriptive summarizing concepts in the ICF regarding people with hearing impairments.

Furthermore, we are not using the ICF as an analytical tool. A comprehensive analysis of hearing impairment and psychosocial effects using the ICF framework is beyond the scope of this book. The purpose of introducing the ICF here is to structure the main chapters in a similar and coherent way. It also signals a common perspective on disability among the authors, that an individual's functioning is an interaction or complex relationship between personal factors and the environment.

References

Andersson Y (2002) ICF from the perspective of deaf people. Newsletter on the WHO FIC 1(1): 4–5.

Davis H (1970) Hearing handicap, standards for hearing and medicolegal rules. In: Davis H, Silverman SR (eds) Hearing and Deafness, 3rd edn. Holt, Rinehart & Winston, New York, p. 255.

Griggs M (1998) Deafness and mental health: perceptions of health within the deaf community. PhD Thesis, University of Bristol, UK.

Kiessling J, Pichora-Fuller MK, Gatehouse S et al. (2003) Candidature for and delivery of audiological services: special needs of older people. International Journal of Audiology 42: 2S92–2S101.

Möller K (2003) Deafblindness: a challenge for assessment – is the ICF a useful tool? International Journal of Audiology 42: S140–S142.

Nordenfelt L (2000) Action, ability and health: Essays on the philosophy of action and welfare. Kluwer, Dordrecht.

Patterson NM (2001) Use of WHO ICIDH-2 for determining aural rehabilitation goals. Professional Research Project, University of South Florida, Directorate of Audiology.

Stephens D (2001) World Health Organization's Classification of Functioning, Disability and Health - ICF. Journal of Audiological Medicine 10(3): vii-x.

Stephens D (2002) Audiological rehabilitation. In: Luxon L, Furman JM, Martini A (eds) Textbook of Audiological Medicine. Martin Dunitz, London, pp. 513-531.

Stephens D, Hétu R (1991) Impairment, disability and handicap in audiology: towards a consensus. Audiology 30: 185-200.

Stephens D, Kerr P (1995) Handicap and its management in the elderly. In: Schoonhoven R, Kapteyn TS, Laat JAPM de (eds) Proceedings of the European Conference on Audiology. Nederlandse Vereninging voor Audiologie, Leiden, pp. 348-352.

Stephens D, Kerr P (2000) Auditory disablements: an update. Audiology 39: 322-332.

Ueda S, Okawa Y (2003) The subjective dimensions of functioning and disability: what is it and what is it for? Disability and Rehabilitation 25: 596-601.

Wade D (2003) Enablement: remarketing socio-medical expectations in rehabilitation. Paper presented to Royal Society of Medicine Wales Meeting 'The power of belief', 12 May 2003.

WHO (1980) International Classification of Impairments, Disabilities and Handicaps. World Health Organization, Geneva, Switzerland.

WHO (1997) International Classification of Impairments, Disabilities and Handicaps - 2 (ICIDH-2). Beta-1 draft. World Health Organization, Geneva, Switzerland.

WHO (1999) International Classification of Impairments, Disabilities and Handicaps - 2 (ICIDH-2). Beta-2 draft. World Health Organization, Geneva, Switzerland.

WHO (2000) International Classification of Impairments, Disabilities and Handicaps - 2 (ICIDH-2). Pre-final draft. World Health Organization, Geneva, Switzerland.

WHO (2001a) International Classification of Impairments, Disabilities and Handicaps - 2 (ICIDH-2). Final draft. World Health Organization, Geneva, Switzerland.

WHO (2001b) International Classification of Functioning, Disability and Health - ICF. World Health Organization, Geneva, Switzerland.

Wood PHN, Badley EM (1978) An epidemiological appraisal of disablement. In: Bennett AE (ed.) Recent Advances in Community Medicine. Churchill Livingstone, Edinburgh.

CHAPTER 4
A common methodology for reviewing the impact of hearing impairment

BERTH DANERMARK, SOPHIA KRAMER AND DAFYDD STEPHENS

Literature search method

In this chapter we give a short description of the literature search on the psychosocial impact of hearing loss on which Chapters 5, 6 and 7 are based. The chapter on deafblindness (Chapter 8) includes a separate description of the literature search dealing with that domain.

We conducted a systematic literature search, using slightly different search tools for different target groups (children, adults and elderly people), and country-specific tools. The search process consists of two major strategies: a manual search and a database search.

- The manual search included searches in audiological journals including the *International Journal of Audiology, Scandinavian Audiology, British Journal of Audiology* and the *American Annals of the Deaf.* Reference lists in books, theses and individual articles were also used. The library of the Royal National Institute for Deaf People and its database was widely consulted.
- The database search was conducted in MEDLINE, ClinPSYC, PsychINFO, Elin@Örebro, EMBASE, CINAHL, Psyc Articles, Eric and Sociological Abstracts, Picarta and Web of Science. We also used Google. Inclusion criteria were: published 1980 or later (occasionally earlier), matching any of the key words shown in Table 4.1. Various specific combinations of these were also used.

Tinnitus and its impact are regarded as a separate field in audiology and are excluded from the present literature search.

With the exception of a few studies published in German, Swedish, Dutch or Danish, we included only literature published in English. This means that some important publications may have been overlooked, but the English literature contains reports of studies in most western European countries.

Table 4.1. Main search items in web searches

Adolescence	Hearing impaired
Childhood	Hearing impairment
Deaf	Hearing loss
Deaf and career	Hearing loss and career
Deaf and family life	Hearing loss and family life
Deaf and psychosocial	Hearing loss and health status
Deaf and quality of life	Hearing loss and psychosocial
Deaf and rehabilitation	Hearing loss and quality of life
Deaf and work	Hearing loss and work
Elderly/older adults	Personality
Emotional disturbance	Presbyacusis
Handicap	

Some important observations can be made, based on the results of the search:

- First, the main body of literature we are dealing with consists of articles reporting findings in empirical studies, quantitative or qualitative. With some exceptions, literature dealing with the issue in more general terms, such as handbooks, encyclopaedias or textbooks, is not included in the review.
- Secondly, a comparison between the manual and database searches reveals that many studies are not found when the databases are searched. Some international audiological journals never appear in the databases we have used. In other instances, it seems that some articles in a journal appear and some do not. Since we have used the most common databases in which one could expect to find the audiological literature, this is an important shortcoming. We have not been able to explore this issue further.
- Thirdly, there is no specific database that is used for audiological literature. In order to find the literature, one has to search in a great number of databases because those most widely used – e.g. MEDLINE and PsychINFO – cover only a minor part of the literature.
- Fourthly, not many databases offer full text articles. This makes the search process costly in terms of time and resources, with many libraries charging increasing amounts for copies of articles.

Bibliography

The result of the systematic literature search is summarized in two bibliographies, one for journal articles and one for books and theses, which are published on the internet (www.gendeaf.org, under 'Psychsocial Group members'). These bibliographies include author names, full article titles, full journal/book titles and years of publication. The overviews are divided into categories representing the different target groups: children and adolescents, working adults and elderly people. The remaining categories include historical books and articles describing theoretical frameworks and models for rehabilitation.

A separate section on the psychosocial impact of deafblindness has been added to the website, as well as a further section on the attitudes of parents of deaf children to genetic interventions.

It is anticipated that the website will be available for the next 10 years, and will be updated regularly. Contributions to this website will be welcomed by the authors of this chapter.

Layout of the chapters

The aim has been to structure the individual chapters according to the ICF framework described in Chapter 3. However, it has not always been easy to fit the reported results into the ICF framework. Outcome instruments usually cover more than one area of the ICF, and are not structured according to the ICF. The presentations start with the psychosocial impact of hearing impairment in children, followed by the impact in working-age adults and finally in elderly people.

In addition, the role of a family history of hearing impairment, where it is documented, is highlighted.

Epidemiology and aetiology

The prevalence of hearing impairment in the three chapters varies considerably, as does the breakdown of such a prevalence by severity. Thus, broadly speaking, the prevalence of permanent childhood hearing impairment is of the order of 0.1-0.2% of the child population, depending on the criteria used (e.g. > 40 dB or > 50 dB). This is discussed at some length by Fortnum (2003). Most studies show prevalence of the order of 0.03% of children having a severe hearing impairment (71-95 dB) with a similar prevalence of profound hearing impairment (> 95 dB).

Impairment in adults is much more common, affecting some 16% of the adult population aged 18-80 years (e.g. Davis, 1995). There is also a major difference in the prevalence as a function of age. If we take a criterion of 40 dB in the better ear (analogous to most recent paediatric studies) the overall adult prevalence is approximately 6%, i.e. 30 times the prevalence reported in children. However, this masks an increase from 0.2% in the 18-30 year age group to 30% in those aged 71-80 years (Davis, 1995).

Moreover, it must also be remembered that many adults seeking help for their hearing problems have a milder hearing impairment and, if the common 25-dB criterion is used, the prevalence rises to 16% of the adult population. Among those over 80 years of age, over 90% of the population has some degree of impairment (Jönsson and Rosenhall, 1998).

The prevalence of profound hearing impairment (> 95 dB) in adults is 0.13% of the population (Thornton, 1986), from which we can assume that three-quarters of adults with such a loss have acquired it. The prevalence of such acquired loss increases particularly after the age of 50 years. It is thus noteworthy that, although such a prevalence of profound loss accounts for some 30% of the hearing impairment found in children, it amounts to only some 2% of that found in adults. Thus, overall, the older the population, the smaller the proportion of the hearing impairment due to prelingual hearing impairment. However, most acquired hearing impairment is of a mild–moderate severity.

Although aetiology is rarely mentioned in the studies, one interesting point emerges. This is that, by most estimates, some 50% of permanent childhood hearing impairment is caused by genetic factors (e.g. Parving, 1996). Recent twin studies have also indicated that some 50% of age-related hearing impairment is genetically determined (Karlsson et al., 1997; Gates, Couropmitree and Myers, 1999).

Beyond this, there are few aetiological parallels between childhood and adult-onset hearing impairment. For example, whereas most childhood deafness caused by genetic factors is severe–profound in the case of recessive conditions and moderate–severe in the case of dominant conditions (e.g. Parving et al., 1996), most clearly defined late-onset genetic disorders in adults are of mild–moderate severity.

Furthermore, one of the commonest genetic disorders in working-age adults is otosclerosis, mainly a conductive disorder, whereas conductive genetic disorders in children are rare. In addition, while childhood genetic impairment is non-progressive in 85% of patients, by definition most late-onset genetic hearing impairment is progressive.

The above figures are largely based on UK populations, but there is increasing evidence that they are representative of the populations of most western countries on which the psychosocial findings described in the next three chapters are largely based.

References

Davis A (1995) Hearing in Adults. Whurr, London.

Fortnum HM (2003) Epidemiology of permanent childhood hearing impairment: implications for neonatal hearing screening. Audiological Medicine 1: 155–164.

Gates GA, Couropmitree NN, Myers RH (1999) Genetic associations in age-related hearing thresholds. Archives of Otolaryngology 125: 654–659.

Jönsson R, Rosenhall U (1998) Hearing in advanced age. A study of presbyacusis in 85-, 88- and 90-year old people. Audiology 37: 207–218.

Karlsson KK, Harris JR, Svartengren M (1997) Description and primary results from an audiometric study of male twins. Ear and Hearing 18: 114–120.

Parving A (1996) Epidemiology of genetic hearing impairment. In: Martini A, Read A, Stephens D (eds) Genetics and Hearing Impairment. Whurr, London, pp. 73–81.

Parving A, France EA, Stephens SDG (1996) Factors causing hearing impairment in identical birth cohorts in Denmark and Wales. Journal of Audiological Medicine 5: 67–72.

Thornton ARD (1986) Estimation of the number of patients who might be suitable for cochlear implant and similar procedures. British Journal of Audiology 20: 221–229.

CHAPTER 5
The impact of hearing impairment in children

DAFYDD STEPHENS

A number of aspects of the impact of hearing impairment in children have been extensively studied, comparing hearing children and those with a hearing impairment. Much of this work has been concentrated on those with severe or profound hearing impairment who largely comprise the Deaf community, but there are increasing numbers of studies dealing with children with milder hearing impairments, including unilateral and fluctuant impairments.

Genetics and deaf parents

The few existing studies on those with genetic aetiologies of their hearing impairment are usually couched in terms of deaf children with deaf parents, and are mainly restricted to children with severe or profound impairments. Deaf children with one or more deaf parents are generally regarded as comprising about 8–13% of deaf children (e.g. Schein and Delk, 1974; Marschark, 1993; Dye and Kyle, 2000). This figure is not usually broken down by aetiological groups but comprises predominantly those with non-syndromal dominant disorders. Such disorders normally give rise to moderate–severe rather than profound hearing impairments (e.g. Parving, France and Stephens, 1996), and in many studies it is not clear how well the groups have been controlled for the level of hearing impairment.

The classic studies by Vernon and Koh (1970) and Conrad (1979) are among the few studies that have attempted to separate out the effects of having genetic aetiology from being a child of deaf parents. Vernon and Koh selected 269 children with a hearing impairment greater than 70 dB with a genetic aetiology for their hearing impairment defined by a 'careful examination of family pedigrees and medical histories'. They separated 79 children with deaf parents from 190 whose parents had normal hearing, and analysed their results separately. They were matched for age, years in school and IQ (Figure 5.1). The group with deaf parents performed significantly better on the four components of the Stanford Achievement Test. The psychological adjustment rated by both teachers and counsellors was the same in the two groups. In addition although the teacher-rated written language was significantly better in the children with deaf parents, their speech-reading and reading ratings did not differ.

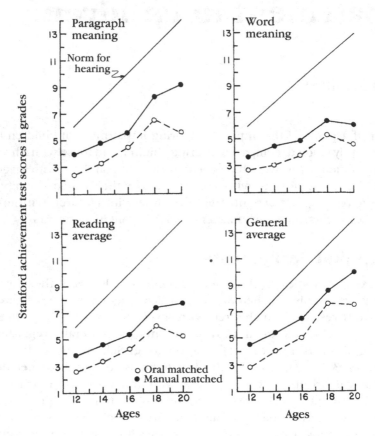

Figure 5.1. A comparison of performance among school students with a genetic hearing impairment. 'Oral matched' is the group with hearing parents brought up orally, matched by age and gender to 'Manual matched', those with deaf parents brought up signing. (From Vernon and Koh, 1970, with the authors' permission.)

Conrad (1979) also separated out the effects of the child having a genetic aetiology, from those of having two deaf parents, by comparing results in these two groups with a group with hearing parents and an acquired aetiology as well as with a group with hearing parents and an unknown aetiology. The groups were age and audiometrically matched.

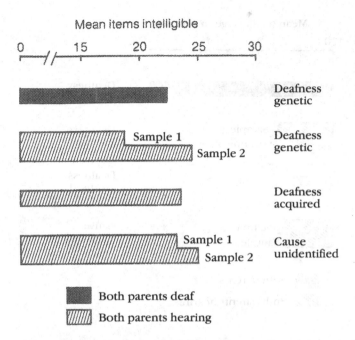

Figure 5.2. Speech intelligibility (numbers: maximum = 40), by cause of deafness and parents' status. (From Conrad, 1979, with the author's permission.)

Figure 5.2 shows the speech intelligibility scores of the four groups, which showed no significant difference. However, when Conrad examined the reading ages of the children, those with deaf parents performed significantly better than the other groups, which did not differ significantly from each other. Similar results were found in a speech comprehension ratio of lip-reading (speech-reading) (Figure 5.3).

Thus the conclusion from these studies is that, in children with a genetic disorders, it is the fact of having deaf parents who communicate with them and interact with them from an early age which is important, rather than the genetic aetiology *per se*.

Kusché et al. (1983), in a further study with groups with deaf parents and with deaf siblings as two 'genetic' groups, found both to have better language achievement scores than non-genetic controls. They argued that this could be attributable to the lower non-verbal IQs in their control groups, which could have been attributable to the aetiological breakdown of the groups. However, in addition, like Vernon and Koh (1970) and Conrad (1979), they did find a significantly better performance in those with deaf parents for vocabulary achievement than in those with deaf siblings but hearing parents.

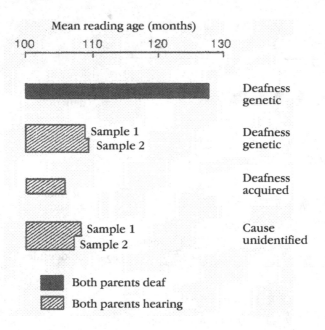

Figure 5.3. Reading age, by cause of deafness and parents' status. (From Conrad, 1979, with the author's permission.)

In addition, borderline differences were found for comprehension ($t = 1.81$; $p < 0.08$) and for language achievement ($t = 1.92$; $p < 0.06$).

Zwiebel (1987), in a study in Israel, compared three groups, one with deaf parents and deaf siblings (DpDs), one with hearing parents and deaf siblings (HpDs) and one with hearing parents and siblings (HpHs). Again he found better cognitive performance in the DpDs group with early use of sign language. He thus also argued that it was early use of sign language rather than genetic factors which resulted in better cognitive performance. There were no differences between the HpDs and HpHs groups.

Differing IQs in different study groups have been a source of controversy (e.g. Conrad and Weiskrantz, 1981; Braden, 1987; Zwiebel, 1987) and have more recently been discussed by Marschark (1993), but are outside the terms of reference of the present chapter.

Early diagnosis

More recent work (e.g. Markides, 1986; Yoshinaga-Itano et al., 1998) has emphasized the importance of early diagnosis and rehabilitation on language development, and more recently on social–emotional development

(Yoshinaga-Itano, 2003). Although these authors did not specifically examine the role of a family history or of having deaf parents, it is certainly possible that having deaf parents facilitates early diagnosis and adjustment, so it remains uncertain from the studies by Vernon and Koh (1970) and Conrad (1979) whether there could be an interaction between these factors.

Most recently Powers (2003), in a study on academic outcomes (General Certificate of Secondary Education [GCSE] results) in English school leavers, found the hearing status of parents to be a significant factor on outcome only in one of two cohorts which he studied, and even this effect vanished on regression analysis. Furthermore, he failed to find an effect of age of diagnosis, although it should be stated that his cut-off points were 12, 24 and 36 months as opposed to the 6-month cut-off used by Markides (1986) and by Yoshinaga-Itano et al. (1998). Furthermore, the fact that the children were in mainstream education will have excluded many children of deaf parents who traditionally prefer their children to attend schools for the deaf.

Impact of aetiological diagnosis

In many studies on the aetiology of childhood permanent hearing impairment, a large proportion falls into the 'unknown' category. Several studies (e.g. France and Stephens, 1995; Parving, France and Stephens, 1996) have indicated that by performing a number of general investigations (e.g. CT scan of the inner ear, urinanalysis, ECG, testing hearing of family members), the size of this group can be significantly reduced. This is important from a psychosocial standpoint.

Thus Meadow (1968) indicated that ignorance of the aetiology can cause great concern among the parents of deaf children. Schlesinger and Meadow (1976) found that, in a residential school for the deaf, 55% of children considered to be emotionally disturbed were listed as 'aetiology unknown' compared with 16% of controls. These authors also found an apparent relationship between a lack of aetiological diagnosis and what they defined as the need for psychiatric treatment in a group of deaf children.

Other factors

It is interesting to note that deaf children with deaf parents usually come from a lower socio-economic level than deaf children with hearing parents (Schein and Delk, 1974; Dye and Kyle, 2000). This would theoretically tend to make them more likely to suffer from poorer educational achievement (Yoshinaga-Itano, 2003).

Marschark (1993) has extensively discussed the development of these differences from early child–parent interactions and bonding, leading to cognitive and linguistic differences between those with and those without deaf parents and between those hearing children with hearing parents. The present chapter does not consider these intermediate steps in any detail, and is limited to the participation restriction and behavioural consequences of such effects.

The coverage of this chapter is restricted to those with simple non-syndromal hearing impairment, excluding those young people with additional disabilities. In addition, the impact of any form of intervention, including audiological (hearing aids, environmental aids, cochlear implants), educational, psychological and medical will not be considered.

In the following sections I consider the impact of the different types and degrees of hearing impairment on each of the various potential aspects of participation and behaviour, and effects on those around the person with the hearing impairment, as outlined in Chapter 3 and derived from the ICF (WHO, 2001). The ICF categories are indicated at the beginning of each section. Under each heading the general psychosocial effects are considered first; then effects specific to those individuals with a family history of hearing impairment are considered within the individual components (shown in italics).

Specific effects – participation restrictions

Mobility – walking, moving and using transportation (d450–489)

There is little information in the literature in this respect. Chermak (1981) among others has discussed the effects of balance disorders on mobility and Gregory, Bishop and Sheldon (1995) report problems related to loss of confidence when travelling, among adolescents with a hearing impairment.

Chermak (1981, p. 350) referred back to studies by Myklebust (1946) and a number of later authors who reported balance and vestibular disorders in deaf children. Indeed, it has been argued (Möller, 1996) that delayed walking in deaf children is one of the best indicators of vestibular involvement. Balance problems affect both children and adults, particularly in the dark where visual compensation is reduced and on rough surfaces where proprioceptive inputs are altered.

This may occur in both non-genetic and genetic disorders, so that the specific impairment of vestibular function is the principal factor causing the problem in this case, rather than whether it is caused by meningitis or by genetic conditions, for example. Indeed, Mazzoli et al. (2001) have shown a great variety in the occurrence of balance disorders with different non-syndromal genotypes.

Gregory, Bishop and Sheldon (1995, pp. 133–139) discuss the problems experienced in travelling by deaf adolescents and give parents' reports indicating that only 22% of their children with a hearing impairment were confident with all forms of transport. Buses seem to pose the most problems, usually because of the lack of understanding shown by bus drivers and conductors. Visual displays in the train service are beginning to reduce problems there, and this is even more true of air travel. The authors also highlight the communication problems of learning to drive, having to listen to the instructions of a teacher often little used to dealing with people with a hearing impairment, or using an interpreter sitting in the car.

Self-care (d5)

Social maturity and self-help has historically been regarded as being delayed in deaf children, but Kricos (1987), considering the methodological implications of the work of Greenberg (1980), argued that this was not necessarily so, given early support for the parents. While Greenberg's groups were small, they were well balanced and comprised only deaf children of hearing parents. These showed no difference from hearing children in the self-help, physical and social scales of the Alpern Boll developmental profile.

Studies by Reeve (2003), in children with mild and unilateral hearing impairments, indicated generally normal performance in many activities although a third of parents, particularly those of children with unilateral impairments, indicated clumsiness. This may be related to balance problems, as has been found in a number of other studies.

Again, there is no evidence of a particular effect of having a genetic disorder in the case of self-care.

Domestic life – acquisition of necessities (d6)

Gregory, Bishop and Sheldon (1995, pp. 123–127) discuss the situation regarding experiences with shopping, banking and obtaining insurance encountered by deaf adolescents. With the increasing number of mainly self-service supermarkets and the introduction of technology, this is becoming a lesser problem than when all commercial transactions were carried out face to face. However, despite this the authors report that 38% need an accompanying person for complex transactions and 11% never shopped alone; 57% needed some parental help for dealing with banking services (although admittedly this study was carried out before the introduction of internet banking).

When they enquired about particular objects purchased, Dye and Kyle (2000) found that, not surprisingly, deaf people were more likely to have videos, home computers and microwaves and less likely to have a CD player than their hearing counterparts. In addition, deaf young people who had a house were more likely to live in terraced accommodation. This may, however, relate to their level of employment and income, and this will be discussed further later.

Interpersonal interactions and relationships (d7)

Informal social relationships – friends (d7405)

In a study on value systems of adolescents with and without a hearing impairment, Bellin and Stephens (2002) asked them to rate 3 out of 9 items (health, love, peace of mind, happy family life, job security, success/money, enjoyment and excitement, leisure and friends) which were the most important for them. Only 39% of the boys but 75% of the girls included friends in these three, compared with 49% and 56% respectively for hearing boys and girls. Thus both were beyond the 95% confidence limits for hearing boys and girls but in opposite directions; boys with a hearing impairment gave friends a low importance rating and girls with a hearing impairment gave them a high importance rating. This illustrates the problems of generalizing within such comparisons. These figures undoubtedly reflect the particular experiences of different groups, given that virtually all of Bellin and Stephens' subjects were in mainstream education.

Various studies (Davis et al., 1986; Gregory, 1998; Ita and Friedman, 1999; Reeve, 2003) have indicated that children with a hearing impairment have difficulty making friends. This is true even of those with mild or unilateral hearing impairments (Davis et al., 1986; Reeve, 2003). Furthermore, children with a hearing impairment find it easier to establish friendships with other children with a hearing impairment and feel more emotionally secure in their friendships with them than with hearing children (e.g. Stinson, Whitmire and Kluwin, 1996). They report lack of friendship and acceptance by hearing children. Thus on the whole they report more loneliness and isolation if they are in mainstream schools than those in residential schools for the deaf (Gregory, 1998).

Further, in a study on friendship by hearing children and children with a hearing impairment in mainstream secondary schools, Markides (1989) found that 51% of hearing-impaired reported their best friend as also being hearing-impaired and 27% hearing. For hearing children, 85% were hearing and only 3% hearing-impaired. When asked why not the opposite group, 15% of the hearing-impaired and 33% of the hearing attributed this to communication difficulties.

To some extent, their preference for deaf or hearing friends depends on their language skills and abilities (e.g. signing vs oral and different levels of oral communication; Gregory, Bishop and Sheldon, 1995) and this is also reflected in reports that hard-of-hearing children tend to have hearing friends and those with severe–profound hearing impairment have deaf friends

(Huttunen, 2000). Similar findings were also reported by Antia and Kreimeyer (2003) in a review of studies of peer interactions. Further, in an interesting study on a group of 29 children with a hearing impairment who were transferred from a mainstream school to a school for the deaf, Brunnberg (2003) found they felt less isolated in the latter environment. They no longer felt themselves to be 'outsiders' at the school for the deaf, and had more self-confidence.

Furthermore, returning to the original findings of Bellin and Stephens (2002), Gregory (1998) reported that all deaf youngsters have problems establishing relationships with members of the opposite sex, with 38% of deaf youngsters over 21 years of age never having had a boyfriend or girlfriend. In particular, 85% of young deaf women were more likely to have partners but only 42% of young deaf men.

There is no definite evidence of the influence of genetic factors on friendships, although deaf children of deaf parents are more likely to attend schools for the deaf than are deaf children of hearing parents.

Family relationships (d760)

One of the main effects of having a hearing-impaired child is that the parents feel a greater responsibility for making social arrangements for these children (Gregory, 1998; Meehan, France and Stephens, 2002). While Meadow (1980) correctly points out that over 90% of deaf children have hearing parents and family, she does not consider the specific implications of this.

Bellin and Stephens (2002) in their survey of attitudes of hearing-impaired teenagers found that they are more likely than their hearing peers to rate 'happy family life' as important than their hearing counterparts do. Unlike the attitude towards friends, this is equally true of boys and girls (63% and 64% respectively).

Meehan, France and Stephens (2002) reported that 26% of all the problems reported by parents of hearing-impaired adolescents on behalf of their children related to the children's overdependence on their parents, their socialization and lack of understanding. Interestingly, in parallel with this, 30% of the problems impacting on themselves as parents come within this context.

Gregory, Bishop and Sheldon (1995) considered whom the deaf child found easiest in terms of relationships and found that for 25% it was the mother, for 20% a sibling and for only 5% the father. Meadow (1980) touched on the tensions which sometime occur between deaf children and their hearing siblings, and this will be discussed further in a later section.

Having a deaf child has little effect on childcare responsibilities and on divorce within the family (Meadow, 1980), although later anecdotal reports do question this conclusion (see Chapter 2).

Parent–infant interactions and relationships (d7600)

Traci and Koester (2003), quoting Meadow-Orlans (2000), comment that this is a field where 'paucity of rigorous studies with deaf populations, in conjunction with frequent inaccessibility of the supports they recommend, weakens the utility of this research as an effective coping resource. . . . Therefore concerns still exist how deafness will affect the child, how the child will affect the family . . .'.

Undoubtedly the development of parent–infant relationships is abnormal in the case of deaf children (Palmer, 2002). Furthermore, this is an area in which most studies have shown major differences between the relationships found between deaf children of deaf parents and deaf children of hearing parents. The argument has been that deaf children are less securely attached to their mothers than are hearing children, although the hard evidence for this is lacking (Palmer, 2002). Marschark (1997) has shown that the strength and stability of mother–child relationships are very much a function of the mother's communicative skills. Thus early diagnosis (e.g. from neonatal screening, Yoshinaga-Itano et al., 1998) can lead to early adjustment by the mother to the child and his or her hearing impairment, whether it is by early amplification, signing or a combination of the two.

Traci and Koester (2003) discuss deafness as a factor interfering with normal psychological development of the children, as a result of their experiences of the world and their social and environmental supports. They also quote Papoušek and Papoušek (1997) as suggesting unfavourable risk factors which may affect mother–child relationships. These are: (1) missed opportunities for initial communication; (2) infant disability leading to discouragement of intuitive parental responses; (3) mismatched style between parent and infant; and (4) prolonged need for infantile preverbal communication. These can all contribute to stresses in the relationship between parents and their deaf child. Such stresses also emanate in part from the grief response experienced by parents of deaf children (Hindley, 2000). This can lead particularly hearing mothers to become intrusive and over-controlling.

Many studies, dating back to earlier psychoanalytic work (e.g. Galenson et al., 1979), have highlighted the different interactions between deaf children of deaf parents and deaf children of hearing parents. However, even in the former group not everything is perfect, with Galenson et al. reporting that their deaf mothers (a sample of only 4!) had introduced early self-bottle feeding with the bottle often positioned so that it faced away from the mother. However, most studies (e.g. Meadow-Orlans and Spencer, 1966) indicated that Deaf infants with Deaf mothers spend more time in coordinated joint attention which, they argue, is one of the most valuable measures of mother–child interaction. In their study, they found that the disparity between deaf children with deaf mothers and those with hearing mothers progressively increased from 9 to 18 months. Furthermore, Matasaka (1992) has demonstrated how deaf mothers of deaf children develop a signed version of 'motherese'.

Overall, although there are many studies that have shown more effective mother–child interactions and relationships for deaf children with deaf parents, none has examined this specifically by aetiological group. Furthermore as Marschark (1997) has shown, this relates primarily to the mother's ability to communicate with the child, and such differences may lessen with neonatal screening and early intervention.

Intimate relationships (d770)

In Gregory's follow-up study (1998; Gregory, Bishop and Sheldon, 1995) she found that young women with hearing impairment were more likely to have a partner than young men with hearing impairment (85% vs 42%). In addition 41% preferred to have a deaf partner as opposed to 14% preferring a hearing partner, with 46% saying that it depended on the circumstances or did not matter. Only one of Gregory's group reported a homosexual relationship. Meadow (1980) found that 70% of deaf parents thought it better for their children to have a deaf spouse, whereas only 17% of hearing parents felt the same way. Schein and Delk (1974) found that 87% have deaf or hard-of-hearing spouses.

Interestingly, again, in the Bellin and Stephens' (2002) study of attitudes of deaf and hard-of-hearing teenagers, both boys and girls were more likely to rate 'love' as an important value than their hearing-impaired counterparts although 42% of the girls rated it as important, compared with 29% of the boys. This followed the same normal gender difference as hearing controls.

More data are available for marriage rates, with Huttunen (2000) finding the likelihood of marriage to be independent of the severity of hearing loss. Dye and Kyle (2000) in the UK found that deaf people were more likely to be married than their hearing counterparts (42% vs 58%), and Jackson and Dilka (2001) in the USA report that only 8% never marry compared with 20% of normally hearing controls. However, both studies report a higher percentage of the Deaf being divorced or separated than hearing controls. Most studies likewise report that, on average, Deaf people tend to marry later than hearing controls (see also Chapter 6).

There are no hard data on the influence of genetic hearing impairment on the intimate relationship, although the attitudinal difference stemming from hearing-impaired parents in favour of choosing a deaf spouse is likely to have an impact on their children's choice of partners.

Sexuality and abuse (d7702)

Surprisingly little has been written on the sexuality of deaf adolescents, beyond largely anecdotal reports (see also Chapter 6). This may be reflected in the reluctance of Deaf and hearing-impaired youngsters to articulate their experience to clinicians and interviewers, although Gregory, Bishop and Sheldon (1995) reported a series of interviews touching on this. Information on different sexual orientations including male and female homosexuality within the Deaf community is lacking, although Swartz (1993) quotes Rainer et al. (1963) as noting an 'apparently higher level of homosexuality among deaf adolescents (roughly 19.6%)'. This was also mentioned by Kallman (1963) who argued that the situation was not being adequately addressed.

Meehan, France and Stephens (2002) attempted to approach the problem of the reluctance of teenagers to articulate any problems in general consequent to their hearing impairment by an open-ended approach to their parents. It was unlikely that parents would provide any pointers in the sexual domain, but they did in fact express some concern about the sexual naivety of their children. Thus 'Has very few hearing peer friends which obviously delays important education in life, such as . . . the dangers of sexual involvement, AIDS, etc'. Such generally delayed development was highlighted by Swartz (1993), who also discussed the concept of delayed learning about interpersonal relationships. However, in interviews with deaf teenagers, Gregory, Bishop and Sheldon (1995) found them to be particularly well informed about HIV/AIDs (p. 203).

Joseph, Sawyer and Desmond (1995) surveyed 134 deaf and hard-of-hearing students at Gallaudet College and found that they had a low level of knowledge of sexual health and a high level of high-risk sexual behaviour, and that they were dependent principally on their peers for information on sexual health, rather than on their parents or school. Elsewhere Fitzgerald and Fitzgerald (1980) have outlined techniques for sexual education programmes in schools for the deaf, but these do not appear to have been widely implemented.

Furthermore, and disturbingly, Joseph, Sawyer and Desmond (1995) highlighted the fact that a quarter of respondents reported that they had been victims of forced sex. A series of important papers on the physical and sexual abuse of deaf and hearing-impaired youngsters has been published by Sullivan and her group from Omaha (e.g. Sullivan et al., 1991; Sullivan and Knutson, 1998; Sullivan, Brookhouser and Scanlan, 2000). Overall their conclusions were that the hearing-impaired teenagers were twice as likely to have been physically abused and 1.4 times as likely to have been neglected as maltreated children without disabilities, whereas sexual abuse was at about 1.3 times the level found in 'normal' children. Risk factors were from members of their own family and also being in a residential institution, such as a residential school for the deaf.

The findings of Sullivan et al. were supported in a Norwegian study of 431 adult deaf people about experiences of sexual abuse in their childhood (Hoem Kvam, 2001). In the Norwegian study the risk ratio that deaf children had been sexually abused compared with their normally hearing peers was about 1.4. They also found that, although girls experience abuse more often than boys, the sex ratio in Norway indicated an even distribution of the sexes among those with hearing impairment. The author also concluded that risk factors (who is the abuser and in what environment) in her findings are in agreement with those from the USA.

In Sweden, Brunnberg (2003) implied that children with a hearing impairment are more susceptible to physical abuse when in mainstream education than in a school for the deaf.

There are no specific references to genetic factors in terms of sexuality, although it should be noted that in the USA and other countries there is frequently a preference of deaf parents of deaf children to send their children to residential school, thus possibly increasing their risk of abuse.

Education (d810–839)

In a paper dating from the beginning of the era of transistor hearing aids, Silverman, Lane and Doehring (1960) commented 'it takes approximately three years to prepare the child for the first grade and a total of from ten to twelve years to complete the eight elementary grades'. Since that time there have been a plethora of studies in the academic performance of deaf children and factors influencing it. Indeed, in a review commissioned by the UK Department of Education and Employment, Powers, Gregory and Thoutenhoofd (1998) surveyed over 300 papers published in the previous 20 years in English-speaking countries. Their review covered the period following Conrad's major study (*The Deaf School Child*, 1979) in the UK as well as a number of key studies by Vernon and others in the USA (e.g. Quigley and Thomure, 1968; Vernon and Koh, 1970; Schein and Delk, 1974). A number of the earlier US studies were reviewed by Kricos (1987) and others, and the more recent publications by Karchmer and Mitchell (2003), among others.

Thus Schein and Delk (1974), in a population-based study, found deaf children overall to be one year below the general educational level; Conrad (1979) found the median reading age of 16-year-olds to be that of normal 9-year-olds; and Gregory, Bishop and Sheldon (1995) found 25% of their adolescent sample to be functionally illiterate, with only one in three a competent reader. They also commented on the greater competence in mathematics than in English, which was consistently found in the studies reviewed by Powers, Gregory and Thoutenhoofd (1998). However, deaf children still perform less well than hearing children even though the difference is less than for English. Most recently Hyde et al. (2003) argued that deaf children doing mathematics are handicapped by the verbal way that the subject is presented and assessed, and argued for more analytical approaches.

The difference between the achievements of deaf children with deaf parents and deaf children with hearing parents has been considered briefly in the introductory section, where it is seen that having deaf parents rather than a genetic aetiology provides a distinct advantage in the educational achievement of the deaf child (e.g. Vernon and Koh, 1970; Conrad, 1979; Kusché et al., 1983; Zwiebel, 1987). More recently, Huttunen et al. (1999) found no difference in academic achievement in Finland by those with and without genetic aetiologies. Braden (1994) found further evidence of a higher IQ in deaf children of deaf parents, who also show greater self-esteem. Toscano, McKee and Lepoutre (2002), in interviews with high-flying students, found their success to be dependent on high parental involvement in early education, higher parental expectations, extensive family communication and high self-image – characteristics common in deaf parents of deaf children (Marschark, 1993). Schroedel and Geyer (2000) have shown that such high fliers obtain better jobs and, interestingly, the deaf in their group succeed better than the hard-of-hearing.

Although a number of studies have shown that those with a less severe hearing impairment achieve better results than those with a more severe impairment (e.g. Järvelin et al., 1997; Powers, Gregory and Thoutenhoofd, 1998), others have not (e.g. Huttunen, 2000). Indeed, a number of studies have indicated quite significant effects of unilateral and mild hearing impairments (Davis et al., 1986; Bess et al., 1998; Bovo et al., 1998; Reeve, 2003) and of long-term otitis media with effusion or glue ear (Haggard, Smith and Nicholls, 2003).

Types of schooling have not been shown consistently to affect the outcome, when other variables have been controlled (Powers, Gregory and Thoutenhoofd, 1998; Karchmer and Mitchell, 2003), even though claims to the contrary have been made (e.g. Lewis, 1996). Indeed in analysing global results obtained by the Gallaudet Research Institute (1996), Karchmer and Mitchell (2003) found the best median results in children in integrated schools followed those in special schools, with those with 'minimal integration' doing least well. There was, however, a very considerable overlap between all the results.

Gregory, Bishop and Sheldon (1995) found that only 7% of their deaf subjects left school with 'A' level examination passes (pre-university examinations usually sat at age 18 years), compared with 22–23% of hearing children. Similar results were found by Dye and Kyle (2000). Powers (2003) also found poor results in GCSE examinations (age 16+) and found that age of onset of the hearing impairment and parental social class were the best predictors of these results.

Although most studies on higher education have been performed in the USA, where there are two famous universities – Gallaudet and the National Technical Institute for the Deaf (NTID) – a few studies have examined attendance at tertiary education in Europe. Thus, for example, Huttunen and Sorri (2001) report that, in northern Finland, only 4% of hearing-impaired youngsters receive tertiary education compared with 22% of all Finns. Dye and Kyle (2000) in the UK found that 6% of young people in the 20–29 age band had degrees or equivalent, compared with 14% of the general population. Huttunen et al. (1999) furthermore found no difference in educational outcome between those with a genetic aetiology and those without.

Furthermore, Danermark, Ström-Sjollund and Borg (1996) found that, compared with hearing students, hearing-impaired Swedish university students tend to be of higher socio-economic status, have more minor medical complaints, feel more lonely or mildly depressed and experience greater anxiety. Danermark, Antonson and Lundström (2001) further found, however, that hard-of-hearing students found more difficulty in coping with changes in intentions and goal regard when in upper secondary education. Academic results and decisions did not depend on the level of their hearing impairment.

In a review of studies on American students, mainly attending NTID, Danermark (1995) had earlier found that the main determinants of dropping out of college were not having attended mainstream school, poor communication skills, and limited goals and commitments.

In terms of attitudes Kafer (1993) found that deaf and hard-of-hearing students perceive grade averages less positively and have less positive attitudes towards school than hearing controls.

Meadow (1980) reported further that most deaf parents preferred to send their deaf children to residential schools where some teachers are deaf and sign language is widely used. However, throughout the world the pattern of schools is changing, with Karchmer and Mitchell (2003) providing US figures for 2000–2001 indicating that less than 25% deaf and hard-of-hearing children now attend special schools.

Overall, in addition to this view of schooling preference, having deaf parents rather than a genetic aetiology per se results in such deaf children performing better than those with hearing parents.

Work and employment (d840–859)

The beginning of work and employment usually signifies the end of childhood and adolescence. The impact of hearing impairment on this will be considered briefly. One of the complications in considering the literature in this field is the changes in the nature of employment opportunities over the past 20–30 years. As long ago as 1981, Vernon highlighted the decline in the manufacturing industries in the developed countries, which had reduced employment opportunities. He particularly emphasized the changed nature of printing, which had traditionally been a source of employment for deaf people. This is discussed at some length in Chapter 6. Since then manufacturing industries have declined and become more automated, with increased work opportunities in the service sector. However, much of the work in the service sector involves communication, which increases the hearing-impaired individual's problems even with the concurrent advances in communicative technology such as the internet and speech recognition techniques.

Among recent studies, Dye and Kyle (2000) in the UK, and Jackson and Dilka (2001) describing the situation in the USA, report higher levels of unemployment in people with hearing impairment than among their hearing peers. Often the unemployment ratio between deaf and hearing is as high as 3 : 1, with Dye and Kyle (2000) finding it higher in women than in men. In addition they report proportionately markedly fewer deaf people in non-manual social groups (professional and white collar). This was also associated with a lower weekly income. It is, however, interesting that they found a much higher proportion of younger deaf people compared with older deaf people in white collar jobs (< 45 years 50%; > 44 years 18% of those in employment). Gregory, Bishop and Sheldon (1995) found that their hearing-impaired young people were more likely to be underemployed than unemployed.

There has been some controversy about the influence of the severity of hearing impairment on employment, with Järvelin et al. (1997) indicating a higher level of unemployment among those with more severe impairment, but Huttunen (2000) finding no such significant effect. Furthermore Danermark, Antonson and Lundström (2001) found that the level of hearing impairment did not determine whether the hearing-impaired youngster went on to employment or to tertiary education. Interestingly, Dauman et al. (2000) found that, among the young impaired group they had followed up, the mean hearing level in the unemployed group was 68 dB as compared with 83 and 88 dB in their two employed groups. Furthermore they found the level of unemployment to be highest among those with non-professional higher qualifications (90%) compared to those with a professional higher qualification (25%) or no higher qualification (36%). How much this is related to the possible involvement and support of the Deaf community is not clear.

Huttunen et al. (1999) appear to be the only group to have examined the impact of aetiology on employment, and then in only a small sample. They found that those with a genetic hearing impairment did not differ from the others in employment status.

Recreation and leisure (d920)

In this category, most of the literature has been concerned with early play by deaf children. Spencer and Deyo (1993) discussed play in terms of Piaget's pre-symbolic and symbolic play. Symbolic play entails various levels of acting out with objects or pretend objects different from reality, and the authors reviewed a range of studies considering the play of hearing-impaired and deaf children within this framework. They found no difference between deaf and hearing 2-year-old children in the frequency of symbolic play, although there was a tendency for deaf children with deaf parents to spend more time on planned object substitution than deaf children of hearing parents, with hearing children in an intermediate position. The authors explained this in terms of the language levels of the children.

Antia and Kriemeyer (2003), in a review of the literature as well as a discussion of their own findings, report that deaf children spend more time in solitary play and less in cooperative play. Children with higher language skills are more likely to involve themselves in cooperative/associative play, but there was no difference between groups in interactions as a whole. In addition, the authors reiterated earlier findings that children are more likely to play with their peers: hearing children with hearing children, etc. Markides (1989) also found this for the playground play of teenage children.

Gregory (1976) reported that, while the same proportion of deaf children play with imaginary friends, they start doing so at a later age. She also reported that while they play with other deaf children as much as with hearing children, they tend to do so separately, each playing his or her own game. She also found that a higher proportion of mothers of deaf children participate in their children's play (88%) compared with mothers of hearing children (66%). Meadow's (1980) finding that deaf children are more indulged by their parents than are hearing children accords with this. She also found that deaf parents of deaf children are more likely to let their children play in the neighbourhood than are hearing parents of deaf children.

In a study on sporting participation by children with various groups of disabilities in Hong Kong, Sit, Lindner and Sherrill (2002) found that children with a hearing impairment were more likely to participate in sports than were other groups. Their motivation was mainly to achieve and receive praise which, the authors argue, is similar to the motivation of most hearing children.

Overall there is a limited literature on deaf children of deaf parents which indicates that, because of their better language skills, they are more likely to participate in symbolic play in ordered sequences. Their parents are more likely to allow them to play with neighbourhood children than are the hearing parents of deaf children.

Religion and spirituality (d930)

Much of the early writing on deaf children emphasized the supportive role of the clergy for the children and their families. The assumption has therefore been that religious beliefs and practice would be higher in such youngsters. However, in their study on deaf adolescents in the UK in the 1990s, Gregory, Bishop and Sheldon (1995) found that only 8% were regular churchgoers and believed in God. Rodda (1970) had earlier found over 70% church attendance by school leavers. Gregory, Bishop and Sheldon argued that this probably reflected the general decline of religious practice in the UK rather than factors specific to the deaf. Figures for deaf adolescents in the USA, where religious practice is much more widespread, are likely to be higher, matching the general population base.

Environmental factors

Within this section discussion is restricted to the elements of support and relationships (Chapter 3) and the attitudes of those around the hearing-impaired child (Chapter 4). Hearing aids, environmental aids (assistive listening devices) and cochlear implants can and do have a major impact on hearing-impaired and deaf youngsters, but are outside the remit of this chapter. Services, systems and policies can likewise have major influences, but are also excluded as they are generally society-specific and again beyond the present terms of reference.

Immediate family (e310)

Parental reactions

Kricos (1987) provided a succinct overview of the reaction of parents to the discovery that their child is deaf. They pass through the stages of the grieving process – denial, anger, bargaining, depression and ultimately acceptance. This can have a major impact on their interactions with the child. Tanner (1980), who discusses the stages of grief in some detail, also outlines ways in which some of the problems can be reduced by appropriate interventions. Punch and Kidd (2001) have recently explored the stages of grief by in-depth interviews and found that the maternal role involved in dealing with a deaf child places considerable strains on families. Furthermore, a high level of conscientiousness on the part of the parents can impede the grieving process. In addition, the parent's experiences of the difficulties encountered by their deaf child can result in chronic sorrow.

Meadow (1980) found that deaf parents of deaf children are less likely to define the finding that their child is deaf as a tragic crisis, and react and interact better with the child because of this. However, in a psychoanalytic study, Galenson et al. (1979) reported that the reaction of a small group of deaf mothers of deaf children was far from normal, with shallow emotional attachment.

Manfredi (1993) described the range of maternal reactions to the recognition of deafness in a child, and to the consequent relationship with the child and with professionals. Parental overall reactions range from maintaining a spontaneous relationship with a child, and taking advice of professionals in a flexible manner, to the responses of those who are transformed into 'an expert's clone', teaching verbal language as if it were an imperative and interacting without spontaneity. From her study of 25 deaf children brought up in an oral programme in Italy, she found that a positive attitude towards deafness and the flexible use of oral communication were the major determinants of positive psychosocial development in childhood.

More recently, concern has been expressed about maternal bonding and the impact of early diagnosis resulting from universal neonatal screening. Yoshinaga-Itano (2003), however, reported no greater parental stresses than with later diagnosis and similar emotional availability to the children as in the case of parents of hearing children. She argued that early diagnosis leads to families resolving their grief earlier.

Calderon and Greenberg (1999) examined predictors of good maternal adjustment and found the two main factors to be social support and maternal problem-solving skills. Earlier, Greenberg (1980) had shown that, in terms of parental attitudes in the Hereford Parent Attitude Survey, there were no differences between parents of deaf children and those of hearing controls. He did, however, find that those with higher communication competence in total communication had more positive attitudes and less stress than those with high oral communication competence.

Little has been published on the effect of the level of hearing impairment on the maternal reaction, but Reeve (2003) indicated that parents of children with a mild sensorineural impairment find it difficult to accept or understand the effects of hearing impairment. Interestingly, this difficulty in acceptance was less in parents of children with equivalent conductive hearing impairments, which Reeve attributed to the frequent presence of other aural symptoms.

Meehan, France and Stephens (2002) asked parents of hearing-impaired teenagers to list the difficulties 'which you have because of your son/daughter's hearing loss'. Of their responses, 56% came in the psychosocial category. Among these, almost half related to the increased dependence (or perceived dependence) of the child on them as parents. Others related to abstract/conceptual limitations and problems explaining psychosexual and emotional concepts.

Overall there appear to have been no studies on the impact of genetic hearing impairment per se, but a number on the impact of having deaf parents. Although these indicate better adjustment to having deaf children, a number of differences from hearing parents of hearing children apparently remain. Further, Young (1995) has shown that families of children raised in a bilingual environment have a more positive coping framework.

Reaction of siblings

Tattersall and Young (2003) report a complex interaction of attempting to maintain normality and feeling more responsibility towards their deaf sibling among six hearing siblings interviewed in depth about their experiences of growing up with a deaf sibling.

Earlier, both Gregory (1976) and Meadow (1980) had reported mainly negative effects of such an experience. Thus, for example, Gregory found that 44% of hearing siblings experience jealousy with regard to their parents' attitudes towards the deaf child, compared with 33% of siblings reacting in the same way to a child with cerebral palsy. However, in Gregory's follow-up study (Gregory, Bishop and Sheldon, 1995) she found that parents reported a good relationship in 57% of cases and a negative relationship in only 9%. Interestingly, relationships seemed to be better for deaf children attending a deaf school rather than for those in mainstream school.

It would be expected that relationships with deaf siblings would be better, but there has been no study focusing on this.

Individual attitudes of people in position of authority (e430)

Gregory, Bishop and Sheldon (1995) discussed some of the experiences of young deaf people with police and social security staff. In general the attitudes were not negative, even though 16% of the deaf youngsters needed help in their interactions.

Stephens, Stephens and Von Eisenhart-Rothe (2000) explored the attitudes of teachers in different parts of the world. Many of the reactions depended upon how much experience the teachers had in dealing with deaf children and the part of the world they came from. Thus teachers questioned in China were more likely to indicate that deaf children should not have the same level of education as hearing children. There were no geographical differences in their responses to the question as to whether children with a hearing impairment would make a lesser contribution to society, although 22% of older teachers felt they would make a lesser contribution compared with 7% of younger teachers.

Personal contextual factors

Table 5.1 shows the listing of personal contextual factors from the ICF (WHO, 2001) which are also discussed in Chapter 3 of this book. In Table 5.1, the sections to be discussed in the remainder of this chapter are shown in bold. The ICF contains only minimal reference to personal contextual factors, so the allocation of particular psychosocial factors to a particular category is inevitably somewhat arbitrary. In some cases the area could be allocated to several different categories, in others it is difficult to define any particular category. However, Table 5.1 may serve as a 'roadmap' for the remainder of the chapter.

Other health conditions – psychiatric disorders

These may be considered as 'other health conditions' in personal contextual factors (see Table 3.10 and Table 5.1).

Table 5.1. A classification of personal contextual factors, based on the ICF (WHO, 2001).

Gender, race, age
Other health conditions
  – **Psychiatric disorders**
Fitness
Lifestyle
Habits
  – **Addictions**
Upbringing
Coping styles
Social background
Education
Profession
Past and current experience
Overall behaviour pattern and character style
  – **Behavioural problems; emotional adjustment**
Individual psychological assets
  – **Personality development; self-esteem; values and aspirations**

Areas of interest in the present context are indicated in bold type

General

The first general population study to consider these was the Isle of Wight study, in the south of England, in which all 11 865 children of compulsory school age were investigated (Graham and Rutter, 1968). They studied the children's psychiatric state using behavioural questionnaires, a systematic interview with the parents and psychiatric examination of the children. While 6.6% of the general child population were found to have psychiatric disorders,15.4% of the deaf children had such problems. Unfortunately for the statistical analysis, this amounted to only two children!

This and later studies have been reviewed by Meadow (1980) and more recently by Hindley (2000). The three largest studies reviewed, with 512, 120 and 294 deaf children respectively, showed prevalences of 31.2, 22 and 22% of psychiatric disorders, while the prevalence in the control populations of hearing children varied from 6.6% to 15.8% in the cited studies, with the prevalence ratios of psychiatric disorders in hearing-impaired to normal children thus ranging from 1.4 : 1 to 3.2 : 1. Thus, overall, there appears to be consistent evidence for a higher prevalence of psychiatric disorders in children with a hearing impairment than in normally hearing children. However, Meadow (1981) pointed out the problem of definitions, in particular the considerable overlap between psychiatric disorders and behavioural problems. An individual child may be classified in different ways according to the professional involved.

The nature of the psychiatric disorders in deaf children has been found to include a higher proportion of social phobias than is found among hearing children (Hindley et al., 1994).

Hindley (2000) has further reviewed risk factors and found communication abilities and family interactions to be key factors. Hindley et al. (1994) found a higher prevalence of psychiatric disorders in schools for the deaf than in hearing-impaired units, although two earlier studies had found the converse to be the case. Furthermore, while Hindley (2000) does not specify it, a combination of family interactions, communicative abilities and attendance at a school for the deaf would suggest that deaf children of deaf parents, among whom communication is generally better from a young age, would be at lower risk. Indeed, in a long-term follow-up of Conrad's (1979) population, Griggs (1998) examined the prevalence of subsequent psychiatric referrals by aetiological group. She found that while 8% of those with an acquired hearing impairment had been seen psychiatrically, only 4% of those with a hereditary cause had had such a referral.

However, after discussing the positive psychological benefits to deaf children of deaf parents, Altshuler (1974) reasonably warned:

The deaf children of deaf parents are not paragons of mental health, and deafness remains a handicap which alters and influences their experience. Nonetheless, the evidence suggests that they do fare better in a number of ways. Clearly this can be laid to the relative lack of parental discomfort with the presence of deafness and the greater freedom and earlier development of communication between parent and child.

Depression

Leigh et al. (1989) examined a group of 102 students at the National Technical Institute for the Deaf, and 112 control hearing students, using the Beck Depression Inventory (Beck, 1967). They found that, while there was a higher prevalence of mild depression among the deaf students (Beck scores 10–18), there was no significant difference between these groups in the context of moderate and severe depression (Beck scores 19 and over). Indeed, for younger children (aged 11–16 years) Hindley et al. (1994) found a paucity of depressive disorders.

Habits – addictions

In the past 10 years the question of alcohol and drug abuse among deaf young-sters has been raised, and even programmes for the treatment and counselling of deaf students discussed (Guthmann and Sandberg, 1995). Overall most studies have indicated that, while deaf students generally have more risk factors for substance abuse, the prevalence of such abuse in the deaf popula-tion is generally lower than in their hearing peers. Thus, Buckley (2001), working with NTID freshmen, found that their abstinence levels from alcohol were high (32% vs 17%) although the prevalence of binge drinking was the same (42%), in the deaf and hearing groups, as was overall marijuana use. Kafer (1993), who reported less alcohol and drug consumption, also stated that her deaf adolescent population reported less intent to use substances.

Recently Wohl and Niehaus (2001) also raised the question of internet addiction in the deaf community, presenting a case history of a Deaf man who had become addicted. They admit, however, that there is no evidence to suggest that the prevalence of such an addiction might be higher among deaf people.

There is no evidence indicating any influence of a family history of deafness on addictive behaviour.

Overall behaviour pattern and characteristic style – behavioural problems and emotional adjustments

Although studies on psychological problems of the deaf date back many decades and there is an extensive literature on the 'psychology of the deaf', the basis of this has been questioned by some authors (e.g. Lane, 2003) and the concept of deaf-wellness has been discussed by Griggs (1998). Lane questioned the concept of 'rigidity, emotional immaturity and behavioural impulsiveness' commonly associated with prelingually deaf children.

However, there are a number of ways in which Lane's analysis can itself be questioned, at least in part. His arguments are mainly from the standpoint of lack of communication between the hearing psychologists and the Deaf community, as well as on the basis of a number of methodological flaws. On this basis, the chief mainstay of the Deaf community might be expected to be the deaf children of deaf parents, who have grown up with sign language. Lane's arguments might be taken to suggest that this group would be those expected to have the most severe psychological problems, and this would be of great relevance to the present discussion of the impact of genetic factors.

Furthermore the question may then be raised of those children with mild or unilateral hearing losses, who have been found by a number of researchers (e.g. Stein, 1983; Smith and Pither, 1993; Reeve, 2003) to have a similar pattern of behavioural problems to children with more severe impairments. In addition, from many studies which they reviewed, Haggard, Smith and Nicholls (2003) highlight a number of behavioural problems in children with persistent otitis media with effusion. This effect becomes less the older the child.

Vernon and Koh (1970) summarized a number of the earlier studies showing better adjustment of deaf children with deaf parents. They also studied a group of children, all of whom had a genetic aetiology, as has been discussed earlier in this chapter. They reported that, while the earlier studies had found that children exposed to sign language by their deaf parents were less disturbed than the oral children, they themselves failed to find a significant difference between the two groups when all had a genetic aetiology. However, they commented that the oral children (of hearing parents) were 'more conforming, passive and compliant' while the signing children (of deaf parents) were 'more questioning and less likely to conform for conformity's sake'. They argued that this behaviour 'does not endear them to teachers and dormitory counsellors'.

Meadow (1980), on the basis of teachers' ratings of deaf children, reported that deaf children of deaf parents were significantly more socially mature than those with hearing parents. She also quoted Vernon's (1969) study indicating that children diagnosed as having a hereditary aetiology were less likely to be severely disturbed, and to have poor psychological adjustment. Thus 10% with a hereditary aetiology had 'poor' adjustment compared with 21% of the whole group. Among children in a residential school for the deaf, she found those with deaf parents to be better in terms of self-image, maturity, independence, sociability and adjustment to deafness.

Studies in Turkey (Polat, 2003) and India (Satapathy and Singhal, 2001) using the Meadows–Kendall adjustment scale have also found better adjustment in deaf children of deaf parents than in those with hearing parents.

Many of the cited studies have shown that deaf children of deaf parents are less likely to have emotional and behavioural problems than deaf children with hearing parents.

Individual psychological assets

Personality development

Some of the comments and reservations expressed by Lane (2003) are equally true in this context in terms of methodological consideration and attitudes towards the Deaf community.

Meadow (1980) reported an increased level of egocentricity and immature responses in deaf youngsters, who tend to be more impulsive and rigid. These descriptors have also been applied to young people with unilateral hearing loss in terms of a sense of embarrassment from their hearing loss (Bovo et al., 1988). Davis et al. (1986) failed to demonstrate any differences between those with a mild hearing loss and those with a more severe loss, in whom they described a tendency to be more aggressive, impulsive and immature.

Some of the aspects of the influence of social isolation, or the self-confidence of teenagers highlighted by Gregory, Bishop and Sheldon (1995), have also been shown by Brunnberg (2003) to be related to the school environment in which they find themselves. Thus some members of a group of hard-of-hearing students developed more self-confidence after being transferred from a mainstream school to a special school for the deaf. Interestingly Gregory, Bishop and Sheldon (1995) found no consistent patterns of personality characteristics in their group of adolescents, commenting that it was 'as might be found in any group of young people'. They further found that only 43% of the youngsters were considered by their parents to be egocentric compared with 55% not so. Equal numbers were considered to be immature and not immature.

There are few hard findings on the personality development of children with deaf parents compared with those of hearing parents, although Galenson et al. (1979) from a psychoanalytical standpoint suggested differences between the personality problems in deaf young children of deaf parents and those with hearing parents.

Self-esteem

Kricos (1987) reviewed studies in this field and found somewhat disparate results. About the same time Warren and Hasenstab (1986) using a picture game with deaf children aged between 5 and 11 years correlated the results with various parental/familial variables and found parental child-rearing attitudes to be the best predictors of self-concept. Unfortunately, only two of the parents in this group were deaf.

Gregory, Bishop and Sheldon (1995) found that most (70%) of their population of adolescents reported that they 'liked themselves' and 55% that they were 'proud of themselves'. However, 64% reported that they would 'like to change themselves' and 42% that they felt 'sorry' for themselves.

Yoshinaga-Itano (2003) found that deaf children diagnosed at an early age were likely to have normal self-concept, although those diagnosed later had lower scores on this scale. Stein (1983) had earlier found children with unilateral hearing impairment to have normal self-esteem. Brunnberg (2003) further found that the confidence of hard-of-hearing children improved and they had more sense of identity when they were in a school for the deaf than when they were in a mainstream school.

No studies appear to have compared deaf children with hearing and deaf parents, although, intuitively, it might be expected that those with deaf parents would be more likely to have higher self-esteem than those with hearing parents.

Values and aspirations

Gregory, Bishop and Sheldon (1995) asked their adolescents 'what do you hope for the future?' and found a marked difference between male and female respondents. Family-related aspirations were listed by 37% of girls but only 9% of boys. Among the boys, the commonest aspirations were work-related (22%) and success/happiness (21%). These compared with 14% and 0% for the girls.

Bellin and Stephens (2002) used a different approach, listing nine potential value areas and asking their deaf and hard-of-hearing adolescents to mark the three most important for them. These results were compared with those obtained from a large group of hearing youngsters of the same age and geographical area.

Table 5.2 shows the results obtained, indicating that, compared with their hearing peers, 'a happy family life' was more important and 'job security' less important for both male and female hard-of-hearing subjects. In addition 'friends' was more important for hearing-impaired girls. Among the hearing-impaired adolescents there was a significant gender effect for 'success/money', more commonly listed by boys, and for 'friends', more commonly listed by girls. Friends do not appear to have featured in Gregory's results but there was a large gender difference in 'success/happiness' with 21% of their male respondents listing this and none of their female respondents.

Table 5.2. Percentage of hearing controls and youngsters with hearing impairment (HI) marking important values (derived from Bellin and Stephens, 2002)

Values	Boys		Girls	
	Controls %	HI %	Controls %	HI %
Health	66	64	70	58
Love	23	29	34	42
Peace of mind	8	4	8	8
Happy family life	34	64*	50	63*
Job security	27	18*	29	4*
Success/money	43	43	24	21
Enjoyment/excitement	29	25	24	21
Leisure	18	14	4	4
Friends	49	39	56	75

*Difference beyond 95% confidence limits.

No results are available from either of these studies in terms of genetic or parental hearing impairment.

Conclusions

Overall there have been only a handful of studies which have compared the psychosocial impact of hearing impairment in youngsters with genetic and non-genetic aetiologies. Where such a genetic hearing impairment has been examined in terms of a parental or non-parental hearing impairment, it has been consistently shown that any difference stems largely from the early communication of parents with the child or children, and the attitude of the parents towards having a deaf child. In all cases the impact of having deaf parents is positive from the standpoint of the child.

It must also be emphasized that most of the studies discussed in this chapter have been concerned with prelingually deaf children. With the exception of the study by Huttunen et al. (1999), all studies reporting the effect of a genetic aetiology or having deaf parents have been concerned with this group with prelingual deafness.

Acknowledgements

The author is most grateful for helpful comments from Mary Griggs. However, any errors are his, and his alone.

References

Altshuler KZ (1974) The social and psychological development of the deaf child; problems, their treatment and prevention. American Annals of the Deaf 119: 365–376.

Antia SD, Kreimeyer KH (2003) Peer interaction of Deaf and hard of hearing children. In: Marschark M, Spencer PE (ed) Oxford Handbook of Deaf Studies, Language and Education. Oxford University Press, Oxford, pp. 164–176.

Beck AT (1967) Depression: clinical experimental and theoretical aspects. Harper & Row, New York.

Bellin W, Stephens D (2002) The value systems of deaf and hearing adolescents. Deafness and Education International 4: 148–165.

Bess FH, Dodd-Murphy SJ, Parker RA (1998) Children with minimal sensorineural hearing loss: prevalence, educational performance and functional status. Ear and Hearing 19: 339–354.

Bovo R, Martini A, Agnoletti M et al. (1998) Auditory an academic performance of children with unilateral hearing loss. Scandinavian Audiology Supplementum 30: 71–74.

Braden JP (1987) An explanation of the superior performance IQs of deaf children of deaf parents. American Annals of the Deaf 132: 263–266.

Braden JP (1994) Deafness, Deprivation and IQ. Plenum Press, London.

Brunnberg E (2003) Vi bytte våra horande skolkamrater mot dova [Hearing impaired children's changes of identity and confidence when changing language in the local environment]. Örebro Studies in Social Work 3. Örebro University, Sweden.

Buckley GJ (2001) NTID freshman deaf college students alcohol and drug use. Journal of the American Deafness and Rehabilitation Association 34: 1–15.

Calderon R, Greenberg MT (1999) Stress and coping in hearing mothers of children with hearing loss: factors affecting mother and child adjustment. American Annals of the Deaf 144: 7–18.

Chermak G (1981) Handbook of Audiological Rehabilitation. Charles C Thomas, Springfield, IL.

Conrad R (1979) The Deaf Schoolchild. Harper & Row, London.

Conrad R, Weiskrantz BC (1981) On the cognitive ability of deaf children with deaf parents. American Annals of the Deaf 126: 995–1003.

Danermark B (1995) Persistence and academic and social integration of hearing-impaired student in postsecondary education: a review of research. Journal of the American Deafness and Rehabilitation Association 29: 20–33.

Danermark B, Ström-Sjollund L, Borg B (1996) Some characteristics of mainstreamed hard of hearing students in Swedish universities. American Annals of the Deaf 141: 359–364.

Danermark B, Antonson S, Lundström I (2001) Social inclusion and career development – transition from upper secondary school to work or post-secondary education among hard of hearing students. Scandinavian Audiology 30 (suppl 53): 120–128.

Dauman R, Daubech Q, Gavilan I et al. (2000) Long term outcome of childhood hearing deficiency. Acta Otolaryngologica 120: 205–208.

Davis JM, Elfenbein J, Schum R, Bentler RA (1986) Effects of mild and moderate hearing impairment on language, educational, and psychosocial behaviour of children. Journal of Speech and Hearing Disorders 51: 53–62.

Dye M, Kyle J (2000) Deaf People in the Community: demographics of the Deaf community in the UK. Deaf Studies Trust, Bristol.

Fitzgerald M, Fitzgerald D (1980) Sexuality and deafness – an American overview. British Journal of Sexual Medicine 7: 24–30.

France EA, Stephens SDG (1995) All Wales audiology and genetic service for hearing impaired young adults. Journal of Audiological Medicine 4: 67–84.

Galenson E, Miller R, Kaplan E, Rothstein A (1979) Assessment of development in the deaf child. Journal of the American Academy of Child Psychiatry 18: 128–142.

Graham P, Rutter M (1968) Organic brain dysfunction and child psychiatric disorder. British Medical Journal 3: 695–700.

Greenberg MT (1980) Hearing families with deaf children: stress and functioning as related to communication method. American Annals of the Deaf 125: 1063–1071.

Gregory S (1976) The Deaf Child and his Family. Allen & Unwin, London.

Gregory S (1998) Deaf young people: aspects of family and social life. In: Marschark M, Clark MD (eds) Psychological Perspectives on Deafness 2. Erlbaum, Mahwah, NJ, pp. 153–170.

Gregory S, Bishop J, Sheldon L (1995) Deaf Young People and their Families: developing understanding. Cambridge University Press, Cambridge.

Griggs M (1998) Deafness and mental health: perceptions of health within the deaf community. PhD thesis. University of Bristol, UK.

Guthmann D, Sandberg A (1995) Clinical approaches in substance abuse treatment for use with deaf and hard of hearing adolescents. Journal of Child and Adolescent Substance Abuse 4: 69–79.

Haggard MP, Smith SC, Nicholls EE (2003) Quality of life and child behaviour. In: Rosenfeld R, Bluestone C (eds) Evidence-based Otitis Media. Decker, Hamilton, Ontario, pp. 401–429.

Hindley P (2000) Child and adult psychiatry. In: Hindley P, Kitson N (eds) Mental Health and Deafness. Whurr, London, pp. 42–74.

Hindley PA, Hill PD, McGuigan S, Kitson N (1994) Psychiatric disorder in deaf and hearing impaired children and young people: a prevalence study. Journal of Child Psychology and Psychiatry 35: 917–934.

Hoem Kvam M (2001) Seksuelle overgrep mot dove barn I Norge. En retrospektiv analyse av situasjonen i barndommen for 431 voksne döve [Sexual abuse of deaf children in Norway. A retrospective analysis of the situation in childhood for 431 adult deaf people]. SINTEF Unimed, Oslo.

Huttunen K (2000) Early childhood hearing impairment, speech intelligibility and late outcome. PhD Thesis, Oulu University, Finland.

Huttunen KH, Sorri MJ (2001) Long term outcome of early childhood hearing impairments in northern Finland. Scandinavian Audiology 30 (suppl 52): 106–108.

Huttunen K, Sorri M, Väyryen M et al. (1999) Educational outcome and employment of Finns with prelingual genetic vs non-genetic hearing impairment – a 15 year follow up. European Work Group on Genetics of Hearing Impairment. Infoletter 6: 36–37.

Hyde M, Zevenbergen R, Power D (2003) Deaf and hard of hearing students' performance on arithmetic word problems. American Annals of the Deaf 148: 56–64.

Ita CM, Friedman HA (1999) The psychological development of children who are deaf or hard of hearing: a critical review. Volta Review 101: 165–181.

Jackson PL, Dilka KA (2001) A psychosocial, educational and economic profile and vocational rehabilitation counselling for the hearing impaired and Deaf. In: Hull RH (ed.) Aural Rehabilitation, 4th edn. Singular, San Diego, CA, pp. 41–55.

Järvelin M-R, Mäki-Torrko E, Sorri MJ, Rantakallio PT (1997) Effect of hearing impairment on educational outcomes and employment up to the age of 25 years in northern Finland. British Journal of Audiology 31: 165–175.

Joseph JM, Sawyer R, Desmond S (1995) Sexual knowledge, behaviour and sources of information among deaf and hard of hearing college students. American Annals of the Deaf 140: 338–345.

Kafer L (1993) Alcohol and other drug attitudes and use among deaf and hearing-impaired adolescents: a psychosocial analysis. PhD Thesis, Ohio State University, USA.

Kallman FJ (1963) The psychiatric problems of deaf children and adolescents. In: The Psychiatric Problems of Deaf Children and Adolescents. NDCS, London, pp. 12–25.

Karchmer MA, Mitchell RE (2003) Demographic and achievement characteristics of deaf and hard of hearing students. In: Marschark M, Spencer PA (eds) Oxford Handbook of Deaf Studies, Language and Education. Oxford University Press, Oxford, pp. 21–37.

Kricos P (1987) Psychosocial aspects of hearing loss in children. In: Alpiner JG, Mc Carthy PS (ed) Rehabilitative Audiology: children and adults. Williams & Wilkins, Baltimore, MD, pp. 269–302.

Kusché CA, Greenberg MT, Garfield TS (1983) Nonverbal intelligence and verbal achievement in deaf adolescents: and examination of heredity and environment. American Annals of the Deaf 128: 458–466.

Lane H (2003) Is there a psychology of the Deaf? Iranian Audiology 2: 16–23.

Leigh IW, Robins CJ, Welkowitz J, Bond RN (1989) Towards greater understanding of depression in deaf individuals. American Annals of the Deaf 134: 249–254.

Lewis S (1996) The reading achievements of a group of severely and profoundly hearing impaired school leavers educated within a natural aural approach. Journal of the British Association of Teachers of the Deaf 20: 1–7.

Manfredi MM (1993) The emotional development of deaf people. In: Marschark M, Clark D (eds) Psychological Perspectives on Deafness. Erlbaum, Hillside, NJ, pp. 49–63.

Marschark M (1993) Psychological Development of Deaf Children. Oxford University Press, New York.

Marschark M (1997) Raising and Educating a Deaf Child: a comprehensive guide to the choices, controversies and decisions faced by parents and educators. Oxford University Press, New York.

Markides A (1986) Age at fitting of hearing aids and speech intelligibility. British Journal of Audiology 20: 165–167.

Markides A (1989) Integration: the speech intelligibility, friendships and associations of hearing-impaired children in secondary schools. Journal of the British Association of Teachers of the Deaf 13: 63–72.

Matasaka N (1992) Motherese in a signed language. Infant Behaviour and Development 15: 453–460.

Mazzoli M, Kennedy V, Newton V, Zhao F, Stephens D (2001) Phenotype-genotype correlation of autosomal dominant and autosomal recessive non-syndromal hearing impairment. In: Martini A, Mazzoli M, Stephens D, Read A (eds) Definitions and Protocols and Guidelines in Genetic Hearing Impairment. Whurr, London, pp. 79–140.

Meadow KP (1968) Parental responses to the medical ambiguities of deafness. Journal of Health and Social Behaviour 9: 299–309.

Meadow KP (1980) Deafness and Child Development. Arnold, London.
Meadow KP (1981) Studies of behavior problems of deaf children. In: Stein LK, Mindel D, Jabaley T (eds) Deafness and Mental Health. Grune & Stratton, New York, pp. 3-22.
Meadow-Orlans KP (2000) Deafness and social change: ruminations of a retiring researcher. In: Spencer PE, Erting CJ, Marschark M (eds) The Deaf Child in the Family and at School. Erlbaum, Mahwah, NJ, pp. 293-301.
Meadow-Orlans KP, Spencer PE (1996) Maternal sensitivity and visual attentiveness of children who are deaf. Early Development and Parenting 5: 213-223.
Meehan T, France EA, Stephens SDG (2002) The use of an open-ended questionnaire with parents of hearing impaired teenagers: an exploratory study. Journal of Audiological Medicine 11: 46-59.
Möller C (1996) Balance function and hearing loss. In: Martini A, Read A, Stephens D (eds) Genetics and Hearing Impairment. Whurr, London, pp. 109-114.
Myklebust H (1946) Significance of etiology in motor performance of deaf children with special reference to meningitis. American Journal of Psychology 59: 249-258.
Palmer S (2002) Psychological effects of hearing impairment. In: Newton V (ed.) Paediatric Audiological Medicine. Whurr, London, pp. 446-463.
Papoušek H, Papoušek M (1997) Fragile aspects of early social integration. In: Cooper PJ, Murray L (eds) Postpartum Depression and Child Development. Guilford Press, New York, pp. 35-52.
Parving A, France EA, Stephens SDG (1996) Factors causing hearing impairment in identical birth cohorts in Denmark and Wales. Journal of Audiological Medicine 5: 67-72.
Polat F (2003) Factors affecting psychosocial adjustment of deaf students. Journal of Deaf Studies and Deaf Education 8: 325-339.
Powers S (2003) Influences of student and family factors on academic outcomes of mainstream secondary school deaf students. Journal of Deaf Studies and Deaf Education 8: 57-58.
Powers S, Gregory S, Thoutenhoofd ED (1998) The Educational Achievements of Deaf Children. Stationery Office, London.
Punch R, Kidd G (2001) Emotional responses of parents of children with hearing impairment: a phenomenological study. Australian Journal of Education of the Deaf 7: 34-42.
Quigley S, Thomure E (1968) Some Effects of Hearing Impairment on School Performance. Institute of Research on Exceptional Children, Urbana, IL.
Rainer J, Altschuler K, Kallman F, Deming W (1963) Family and Mental Health Problems in Deaf Population. New York State Psychiatric Unit, New York.
Reeve KJ (2003) Children with mild unilateral hearing impairment: current management and outcome measures. PhD Thesis, University of Nottingham, UK.
Rodda M (1970) The Hearing Impaired School Leaver. University of London Press, London.
Satapathy S, Singhal S (2001) Predicting social-emotional adjustment of the sensory impaired adolescents. Journal of Personality and Clinical Studies 17: 85-93.
Schein JD, Delk MT (1974) The Deaf Population of the United States. National Association of the Deaf, Silver Spring, MD.
Schlesinger HS, Meadow KP (1976) Emotional support for parents. In: Lilles DL, Trohanos PL, Goin KW (eds) Teaching Parents to Teach. Walker, New York, pp. 35-47.
Schroedel JG, Geyer PD (2000) Long term career attainments of deaf and hard of hearing college graduates: results from a 15 year follow-up survey. American Annals of the Deaf 145: 303-314.

Silverman SR, Lane HS, Doehring DG (1960) Deaf children. In: Davis H, Silverman SR (eds) Hearing and Deafness, 2nd edn. Holt, Rinehart & Winston, New York, pp. 413-451.

Sit CHP, Lindner KJ, Sherrill C (2002) Sport participation of Hong Kong Chinese children with disabilities in special schools. Adapted Physical Activity Quarterly 19: 453-471.

Smith WR, Pither RE (1993) Long term follow up of children with mild hearing impairment: pre- and post intervention. Journal of the British Association of Teachers of the Deaf 17: 99-103.

Spencer PE, Deyo DA (1993) Cognitive and social aspects of deaf children's play. In: Marschark M, Clark MD (eds) Psychological Perspectives on Deafness. Erlbaum, Hillside, NJ, pp. 65-91.

Stein DM (1983) Psychosocial characteristics of school-age children with unilateral hearing loss. Journal of the Academy of Rehabilitative Audiology 16: 12-22.

Stephens D, Stephens R, Eisenhart-Rothe A Von (2000) Attitudes towards hearing impaired children in developing countries - a pilot study. Audiology 39: 184-191.

Stinson MS, Whitmire K, Kluwin TN (1996) Self-perceptions of social relationships in hearing-impaired adolescents. Journal of Educational Psychology 88: 132-143.

Sullivan PM, Knutson JF (1998) Maltreatment and behavioural characteristics of youth who are deaf and hard of hearing. Sexuality and Disability 16: 295-319.

Sullivan PM, Brookhouser PE, Scanlan JM, Knutson JF, Schulte LE (1991) Patterns of physical and sexual abuse of communicatively handicapped children. Annals of Otology, Rhinology and Laryngology 100: 188-194.

Sullivan PM, Brookhouser P, Scanlan J (2000) Maltreatment of deaf and hard of hearing children. In: Hindley P, Kitson N (eds) Mental Health and Deafness. Whurr, London, pp. 149-184.

Swartz DB (1993) A comparative study of sex knowledge among hearing and deaf college freshmen. Sexuality and Disability 11: 129-147.

Tanner DC (1980) Loss and grief implications for the speech-language pathologist and audiologist. ASHA 22: 916-928.

Tattersall HJ, Young AM (2003) Exploring the impact on hearing children of having a deaf sibling. Deafness and Education 5: 108-122.

Toscano RM, McKee B, Lepoutre D (2002) Success with academic English: reflections of deaf college students. American Annals of the Deaf 147: 15-23.

Traci M, Koester LS (2003) Parent-infant interactions. In: Marschark M, Spencer PE (eds) Oxford Handbook of Deaf Studies, Language and Education. Oxford University Press, Oxford, pp. 190-202.

Vernon M (1969) Multiply Handicapped Deaf Children: medical, educational and psychological considerations. Washington Research Monograph for Council for Exceptional Children.

Vernon McK, Koh SD (1970) Early manual communication and deaf children's achievement. American Annals of the Deaf 115: 527-536.

Warren C, Hasenstab S (1986) Self concept of severely to profoundly hearing impaired children. Volta Review 88: 289-295.

Wohl AB, Niehaus M (2001) Internet addiction and the deaf community: a case study on risk, treatment implications and the need for more research. Journal of the American Deafness and Rehabilitation Association 35: 1-7.

WHO (2001) International Classification of Functioning, Disability and Health - ICF. World Health Organization, Geneva, Switzerland.

Yoshinaga-Itano C (2003) Universal newborn hearing screening programs and developmental ourtcomes. Audiological Medicine 1: 199–206.

Yoshinaga-Itano C, Sedley AL, Coulter DK, Mehl AL (1998) Language of early and later-identified children with hearing loss. Pediatrics 102: 1161–1171.

Young A (1995) Family adjustment to a deaf child in a bilingual bicultural environment. PhD Thesis, University of Bristol, UK.

Zwiebel A (1987) More on the effects of early manual communication of the cognitive development of deaf children. American Annals of the Deaf 132: 16–20.

CHAPTER 6
A review of the psychosocial effects of hearing impairment in the working-age population

BERTH DANERMARK

The aim of this chapter is to review some of the literature on the consequences of hearing loss for people of an economically active age, here called the working-age population, although, as I shall show, not all of them are working. However, it is not possible to exactly define the boundaries in terms of age since this information is not always given in the literature and the definition of 'working age' differs between studies. When possible and meaningful, we also try to report the findings focusing on different subgroups: deaf and hard-of-hearing, and sometimes also early or late onset. However, in many articles no information is provided regarding the degree or time of onset of the hearing loss. 'Deaf' and 'hard-of-hearing' are often lumped together and, as reported in *The Deaf Canadian Magazine* (Editorial, 1981), 'There has been a tendency on the part of hearing people to lump the deaf and the hard-of-hearing together into an unnatural and unwieldy conglomerate, labelling it with a bland and nebulous term: "hearing-impaired." The result has been confusion . . .' (in Laszlo, 1994, p. 248). The scientific community has to some extent contributed to this confusion.

The chapter is mainly structured according to the ICF concepts. However, it is sometimes difficult to separate different aspects of psychosocial consequences according to this classification. As will be clear, there are also aspects of the ICF that are of less relevance or are not highlighted in the literature.

As the social model of disability has developed and become more and more applied, the focus has shifted from individual deficits to environmental barriers. This has implications when using the concept of 'consequences'. For instance, when analysing forced early retirement, a common phenomenon among hearing-impaired people, one has to consider many factors at different levels; biological, psychological, socio-economic and cultural. Therefore, when talking about consequences of hearing impairment, we cannot *a priori* state that there is a one-dimensional causal relationship between hearing impairment and psychosocial factors. It is important not to locate the causes in the impairment itself when they are caused by factors at other levels, e.g. social barriers.

In the literature there are also reports on consequences reported by significant others, mainly family members but also co-workers and other people in close relationship to the person with a hearing impairment. Some of these findings are also described and discussed in this chapter.

Communication (d310–d369)

Deafness

Much of the research and literature on communication and deafness is contextual, for instance communication in work settings or in classrooms, and will be dealt with under separate headings in this chapter. Here we will point only to some research that addresses communication from a more general psychosocial perspective. There is also much literature focusing on the issue of sign language, but this topic is not dealt with in this book.

On the basis of many years of research, Foster (see, for example, Foster and DeCaro, 1991; Foster, 1992, 1998) highlights some of the major causes of poor communications between deaf and hearing people. Although Foster (1998, p. 123) stresses that not all communication is impaired since some deaf people are very orally skilled and some hearing people know sign language, it is very often the case. One cause of impaired communication is when the direct contact is broken because the deaf person uses an interpreter (broken eye contact) or uses writing, which is time-consuming and often inappropriate. Another is when the communication is stalled, which occurs when a deaf person tries to use her voice but cannot make herself understood, or when a hearing person cannot be understood despite trying to speak clearly and loud. A third cause is misunderstanding. One participant thinks that the conversation was successful, but finds out later that it was not. The impact of the unsuccessful communication is most often negative, especially the long-term consequences. Furthermore, it affects both the deaf and the hearing person. Foster mentions teasing and ridicule, a feeling of loss and isolation and, in a broader sense, a social rejection by hearing people with withdrawal and isolation as consequences. Impaired communication produces different types of stereotypes and assumptions about deaf people. Among them is the concept that the deaf person wishes to be alone or prefer to be only with other deaf people. A response to this is the development of social networks among deaf people.

Foster and MacLeod (2003) described a number of strategies that deaf people use in order to facilitate the communication with hearing people in work settings. These strategies are: flexibility; taking control of the communication event or creating (engineering) the environment to enhance communication; being in a position of authority (people need to communicate with you); identifying and cultivating key informants; finding a balance.

Hard-of-hearing

Communication problems among hard-of-hearing people are of a different nature from those among the deaf. Congenitally deaf people have their own language, and face communication problems mainly in interaction with people who do not know sign language. Hard-of-hearing people are almost always confronted with communication problems. Whenever they are in less than ideal listening conditions, they experience difficulties to various degrees.

Many studies include a discussion of the consequences of hearing loss for communication. It is obvious that communication problems related to hearing impairment are among the most serious consequences. Communication problems in turn result in, for example, restricted social involvement, stress, anxiety and negative self-image (Hétu et al., 1988). In this sense communication is *the* mediating factor between hearing impairment and psychosocial consequences.

A number of studies focusing on communication strategies are reported elsewhere in this chapter, but we do not discuss studies that focus on verbal communication behaviour, e.g. fluency or repair strategies (see, for example, Gagné and Wyllie, 1989; Caisse and Rockwell, 1993; Tye-Murray and Witt, 1996).

Since communication problems are extremely common and restrictive for practically all social activities, communication is explicitly or implicitly commented upon in other sections of the chapter.

Interpersonal interactions and relationships (d7)

Early-onset deafness

Family life (d760)

Family life is a broad concept and covers many aspects, some of which have been targets for research. Moores, Jatho and Dunn (2001), in an overview of the 21 articles addressing topics concerning families with deaf members published in *American Annals of the Deaf* in 1996–2000, found four main categories: interaction and involvement; support service; stress and coping; and decision-making (cochlear implants and communication modes). With regard to interaction and involvement, these authors noted that, according to the literature, it seems when addressing this issue that the focus had changed from the mother–child dyad only, to include other 'significant others' including members of the deaf community. Some of the studies emphasized the importance of the dynamics of the extended family, but still it is the mother who is the primary caregiver and the most important person in the child's environment. In a Turkish study (Fisiloglu and Fisiloglu, 1996) the authors concluded that families of deaf and hard-of-hearing children adjusted quite well and this conclusion is also supported in a US study (Mapp and Hudson, 1997). However, the results are not unequivocal. Other studies reported stress among the parents and a need for support in coping with raising a deaf child (Lampropouplou and Konstantareas, 1998; Calderon and Greenberg, 1999; Koester and Meadow-Orlans, 1999). Moores, Jatho and Dunn (2001) concluded that 'in general, it appears that most parents are resilient. The presence of a deaf child in a family with hearing parents may cause stress, but stress is a fact of life' (p. 250).

Another approach to this issue is found in P-I Carlsson, B Danermark and E Borg (2004) who investigated civil status and the number of children born among deaf people in two Swedish regions, one with a strong deaf community and the other without. The authors concluded that, among deaf people with early-onset deafness, the proportion who were married was lower than among the general population despite the region they lived in. However, it is interesting to note that in the region with a strong deaf community the average number of children of deaf women was significant higher (1.33) than for deaf women in the region with a weak deaf community (1.16). However, in both regions the numbers were lower than among the general population (1.63 and 1.55, respectively). The finding that deaf women give birth to fewer children, especially if the deafness is congenital, is also true in the USA (Jackson, 1982; Schein, 1982) and in the UK (Middleton, 1999). The authors also found a difference regarding divorces. In the region with a strong deaf community the divorce rate among deaf people was equal to that in the general population, but in the region with a weak deaf community the divorce rate was significant lower. The results indicate the importance of living in a region with a strong deaf community, but for establishing the nature of this influence on family life further studies are required.

Late-onset deafness

Family life (d760)

As described above, when a family member acquires a severe hearing loss it puts much pressure on the family. Sometimes it affects the relationships in the family in a negative way (Meadow-Orlans, 1985; Jones, Kyle and Wood,

1987; Kyle and Wood, 1987). It is worth noting that we have not found any study focusing on the significant others of a person with late-onset deafness. In the studies mentioned below that focus on the spouse's view, the partner is hard-of-hearing. Although there are a number of studies that contain information about the changing family relationships, our knowledge of this issue is very limited and is mainly based on information from the deafened themselves. This is a pitfall, since the view of the significant others seems to be very important. Kyle (1985) emphasized that it is the family adjustment that determines whether the acquired deafness will be successfully coped with or not. It is therefore an extremely important issue, although little studied in the literature.

Some studies report a higher divorce rate among late-deafened adults than among non-disabled people (Glass and Elliott, 1992). Luey (1980) found that half of her deafened subjects had divorced. However, there is not much empirical support for a higher divorce rate, and the results should be interpreted with great caution. Further research is needed before we have any firm knowledge of the relationships between acquired hearing loss and divorce.

There are reports on oppression, exclusion and isolation within the family. The overall problem is related to problems in communication. If the deaf person learns sign language, it seems to be uncommon for the significant others to do this (Aguayo and Coady, 2001). Even if some of the family members do learn sign language, the deaf person's communication needs are often overlooked, resulting in the person reporting a feeling of being excluded from family interaction. This exclusion results in, for example, being left out of discussions and decision-making at home. In the Belfast study (Cowie and Stewart, 1987) 60% of the sample 'felt that their deafness caused stress in the home and that this stress affected their lives badly or very badly' (p. 145). This was noted whatever the level of hearing or time of onset.

Hard-of-hearing

Family life (d760)

Some studies address the consequences experienced by the significant others. One of the most common reported consequences is related to communication and verbal interaction. Stephens, France and Lormore (1995) administered a problems questionnaire to significant others, asking them to list the problems they themselves experienced as spouses and which problem the patient was experiencing. The results indicated that the psychosocial problems dominated and, among them, frustration was the most common, reported by both the significant other and the patient. In most cases the problems stemmed from communication breakdowns and the most commonly listed problem by the significant other was 'Having to repeat' (50%).

Due to the reduced hearing capacity and the inability to cope with these misunderstandings from both sides, reduced frequency of interaction and narrowing of the content of communication were reported in a study conducted among workers with occupational hearing loss. The authors concluded that this would lead to 'devastating effects on family life and intimate relationships' (Hétu, Getty and Quoc, 1995). Among the disadvantages found were the need for a quiet period after a workday, loud TV and radio listening, and loud voice. Tension, stress, anger and resentment were the result of these inconveniences (p. 506). Since these difficulties create serious problems for the family and, as mentioned above, the support of the family is extremely important for the success of the rehabilitation, there is a great need to include the whole family in the rehabilitation process (see also Hétu et al., 1988).

In a qualitative study based on in-depth interviews of 10 women, Hallberg and Barrenäs (1993) and Hallberg (1999) found that there were two important aspects of living with a man with noise-induced hearing loss: the husband's reluctance to acknowledge the hearing difficulties, and the consequences for the intimate relationship. By combining these two aspects, the authors were able to describe four qualitatively different strategies used by the spouse. One is called 'Co-acting', where the spouse plays the game and does not admit any impact of the hearing loss. Another is 'Mediating' (controlling, navigating, advising) and is based on the fact that the wife does not admit the consequences but refuses to play the game. In the third strategy, 'Minimizing', she plays the game but at the same time admits that there are problems, and in the last one, 'Distancing', she both admits the problems and refuses to play the game. However, there are no further studies that can answer the question as to whether these strategies are stable, if the spouse constantly switches between them, how a population of spouses of husbands with noise-induced hearing loss are distributed among the different strategies, and so forth.

Major life areas

Work and careers (d840–859)

There is a substantial body of literature on hearing loss and work, but as Hétu, Getty and Quoc (1995) point out 'No systematic inquiry on hearing disabilities and handicap situations resulting from OHL [occupational hearing loss] in the workplace has been conducted.' (p. 497). The same is true for other categories of hearing loss. In this section we give some examples of the research that has been conducted, mainly in Canada, the USA and Sweden and, to some extent, in the UK. From a disability perspective there are some important differences between these countries that make transcultural comparisons difficult: the features of the labour market, legislation and the dominating norms and values in society.

Early-onset deafness

We begin with some examples of studies focusing on prelingually deaf people. The first consequence to be addressed is whether this group of deaf people has a higher rate of unemployment than the population in general. Among some authors (e.g. Scherich and Mowry, 1997) there seems to be a general assumption that the unemployment rate among deaf people is comparable with the unemployment rate among people with disabilities in general. After stating that 'the rate of unemployment for working age people with disabilities has changed very little – down to 31% in 1994 from 33% in 1986', referring to Holmes (1994), Scherich and Mowry turn to discuss the situation for deaf people without presenting any unemployment figures for them. However, it seems that the unemployment rate among deaf people is comparable with the unemployment rate among 'people with disabilities' or at least significantly higher than among non-disabled people, in the USA and some EU countries (see Chapter 5), but this is not the case in Sweden where the unemployment rate among hearing-impaired people, is about the same as for the population in general. The fundamental difference between deaf people and hard-of-hearing people, on the one hand, and a general population, on the other, is not in the rate of employment – which is about the same across the groups, on average about 75% for the population aged 16–64 years – but that among the groups with hearing impairment a significantly higher proportion is forced into early retirement. Taking early retirement is more than twice as common among deaf and hard-of-hearing people as among the general population (about 12% compared to 5.4%). On the other hand, about 12% of the general population are in education compared to only about 5% of deaf and hard-of-hearing people (SOU, 2001, p. 56). This structural difference is illustrated in Figure 6.1. However, there are some differences between different age groups, indicating that among younger hearing-impaired people there is an over-representation of unemployment (see below). It has also been suggested that underemployment is a more serious problem than unemployment among deaf people (Backenroth, 1995).

Another issue is attitudes to different types of jobs. This subject has been investigated around the world over the last 20 years. Studies have been conducted in the UK, Israel, Italy, South Africa, the USA, India and Sweden (for an overview see DeCaro, Mudgett-DeCaro and Dowliby, 2001). The latest

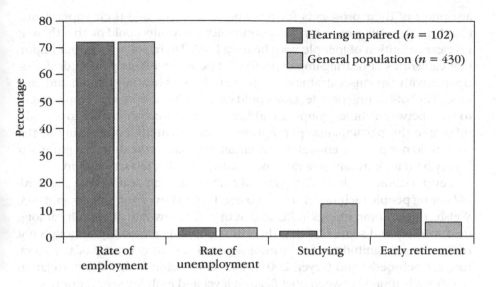

Figure 6.1. Structural differences (percentage) with regard to economic activities between a hearing-impaired population and a general population aged 20–64 in Sweden, 2001.

reported study was done in Sweden by DeCaro and colleagues (2001). The authors conclude that 'surprisingly, the results obtained were remarkably consistent in regard to the expressed advice given to deaf and hearing people to train for various occupations' (p. 51). The advice was partly based on considerations of communication and safety factors. These findings led the authors to ask whether deafness could be a 'cultural homogenizer in regard to attitudes toward careers' (p. 51).

Most of the literature in the field of hearing impairment and employment is about employment experiences in terms of integration/isolation, career advancement, mobility and different types of barriers. Some of the findings can be summarized using Backenroth's words: 'isolation, a lack of feeling of community, a lack of feedback, unconfirmed identity, insufficient inspiration from work, missing important information given at work, missing opportunities for further training, a lack of respect from hearing associates, psychic fatigue and psychic imbalance' (1995, p. 85). Although some of Backenroth's findings are found in many other studies (more recently in Scherich and Mowry, 1997; see also Foster, 1987, 1992) the question is whether this is too negative a picture. Schroedel and Geyer (2001), among others, have challenged this view. After a review of the literature, they conclude that most deaf people report that they are satisfied or very satisfied with their jobs. They write, for instance, that 'most respondents were satisfied with various attributes of their prospects for promotion, careers, and their supervisors' (2001, p. 41). One reason for these contradictory results could be that there is no clear definition of 'people with hearing loss'. There are at least four important categories of hearing-impaired people: people with early-onset deafness, people with late-onset deafness, early-onset hard-of-hearing people and late-onset hard-of-hearing people. One could expect satisfaction with employment to vary between these groups. In addition, the degree of hearing loss might influence the participants' perception of employment. Since many of the studies do not provide enough information to separate the different groups, it is very hard to draw any general conclusions regarding job satisfaction.

Several studies address occupational mobility among deaf people and hard-of-hearing people (Schroedel, 1976; Foster, 1987; Mowry and Anderson, 1993; Welsh, 1993). Some studies indicate that there is a low rate of mobility among deaf workers and some find that there is occupational mobility, although not of the same magnitude as for hearing workers (for an overview of the literature see Schroedel and Geyer, 2001). One conclusion is that the correlation traditionally found between qualification level and mobility seems not to exist among deaf people. Some reasons for the relative lack of mobility, or the lower mobility of deaf workers regardless of education level, are that there are no established career paths (Welsh and Walter, 1988) and that these people have poor reading skills (Schroedel, 1976; Allen, 1986). However, many of these conclusions are based on research in the USA before the implementation of the Americans with Disability Act 1990 and the Workforce Investment Act of 1998. The nature of the labour market has also changed radically during the last two decades, and the results of studies conducted during the 1980s are probably not valid for the situation at the beginning of this century.

One of the few studies that addressed occupational mobility in the late 1990s is Schroedel and Geyer's (2001) longitudinal study of 240 deaf and hard-of-hearing alumni who graduated during 1983–1985 from 47 2-year and 4-year courses at colleges and universities. In 1989, 490 alumni responded to a questionnaire addressing these issues and in the 1999 survey 240 of them answered a new questionnaire. This is a drop-out rate of nearly 50%, which makes it very difficult to draw any general conclusions about occupational mobility among this group, but it does provide many interesting findings for those who answered the questionnaire. The authors do not discuss the implications of the drop-out on the results, e.g. that those with less successful occupational careers were more reluctant to answer the questionnaire than those who were successful, but they point to another limitation, that the result might not be applicable to deaf workers without college education. Furthermore, there is no reference group that can illuminate whether those who answered the questionnaire differed from their normally hearing peers regarding promotion and career and, if so, to what extent. Despite these shortcomings, it is interesting to note that only 45% of the respondents had been promoted since 1995. Length of tenure, supportive supervisors and hearing ability were factors that increased the probability of being promoted. In contrast to other findings, Schroedel and Geyer (2001) did not find that educational level, gender or performing as a supervisor correlated with promotion. The lack of correlation between qualification level and promotion could be a result of all the respondents being college graduates. It is also important to note that about 75% were satisfied with their careers, with their prospects for promotion and with their supervisors. It is also noteworthy that 'white-collar employees were more likely to be promoted than blue-collar workers' (p. 41).

The importance of education is further indicated by a study of El-Khaime (1993) among 490 deaf and hard-of-hearing people, which found that deaf people who had a college or university degree had a better position on the labour market than deaf people with only a high-school qualification. For instance, the unemployment levels were much lower for those with a higher degree than for those without.

Late-onset deafness

As mentioned above, it is not always possible to distinguish between pre- and postlingually deaf people in the literature. However, in some reports we have been able to single out studies that focus on postlingually deaf people. In relation to employment there is an important difference between pre- and postlingually deaf people. Prelingually deaf people choose an educational and employment career based on the fact that they are deaf, but this is not the case for most deafened adults, whose career is generally usually based on the fact that they belong to the hearing world. Together with the often severe individual effects described above, these people face a situation in which they are forced to make major career changes. In a study reported by David and Trehub (1989), 16 of 25 subjects in the study changed careers after the onset of hearing loss.

Among the studies we have come across, only a few deal with the psychosocial work environment for adults with severe–profound hearing impairment (Ringdahl and Grimby, 2000). The authors concluded that this group constituted a risk group in terms of health-related quality of life. Among this population, only three used sign language. Although most of them found their job stimulating, many reported feelings of fatigue and being alienated and that their efforts to communicate led to exhaustion both during working hours and after work, with the family. However, among this group, those who were working full-time ($n = 35$) scored better on most dimensions (this is in accordance with the result presented by Galán et al., 2000). There were no differences regarding pain, emotional reactions and sleep disturbance. They also note that personal harmony among those full-time workers was about the same as among the normally hearing reference population. This indicates either the great importance of having a full-time job, or that the results are biased because the study subjects might constitute an élite sample, or that the sample was too small and the result might not be confirmed in a larger population. The authors consider both possibilities.

Hard-of-hearing

There is some clear evidence that hearing-impaired people constitute a very vulnerable group in the labour market. Parving and Christensen (1993) report that 30% of hearing-impaired people 20–35 years of age in their study (all living in the city of Copenhagen) were unemployed, compared to 12% among all in that age group in Denmark. They also noted that there was no difference between those with a congenital/early onset (before 2 years of age) and subjects with acquired hearing loss after 2 years of age. These findings are also supported in a Finnish study by Huttunen et al. (1999). They reported that in a group of 51 people born in Finland in 1965–1979, all with sensorineural, non-syndromal prelingual hearing impairment, the unemployment rate was more than double among these compared to an age-matched group. They also concluded that it seems to be the severity rather than the aetiology that is important.

As mentioned above, in Sweden hard-of-hearing people in the 20–64 age group are very much over-represented in the group with early retirement, 12.0% compared to 5.4% among the general population (Danermark and Coniavitis Gellerstedt, 2004b). There are furthermore indications that hearing-impaired people are over-represented in the group taking long-term sick leave.

A Finnish study of educational outcomes and employment among hard-of-hearing people up to the age of 25 years (Järvelin et al., 1997) indicates the same situation for them. However, the authors make an important qualification: the unemployment rate was higher (odds ratio 1.9, i.e. twice as high) only among those with a clinically significant hearing loss (when the pure-tone average exceeds 25 dB in the better ear). This group constituted 14% of the total hard-of-hearing group in the study. For those with less hearing loss (86%) there was no difference in the employment rate compared to the normally hearing reference group.

There are many barriers and obstacles to prevent integration into work for this group of employees. Laroche, Garcia and Barette (2000) found in their investigation that hearing-impaired people, audiologists and employers shared some general opinions about the barriers but they also emphasized different conditions or attributes regarding social integration. The greatest barriers mentioned were noise, number of speakers, attitudes of the interlocutors, awareness of the disorder and expectations relating to levels of productivity (p. 75). However, different categories sometimes emphasized different barriers. Employers were the only group that mentioned the realities of the job market as a barrier. The hearing-impaired people did not mention communication tasks and productivity as barriers, but these two factors were mentioned by both audiologists and employers. This divergence is interesting, since both type of barrier can be assumed to play an important role in work integration. The result is also contradictory to the findings of Hétu, Getty and Quoc (1995) who reported, on the basis of a questionnaire, that hard-of-hearing people have communication difficulties whenever background noise is present. Furthermore, there is also a risk of their not appreciating an emergency when working in dangerous situations (p. 503). The hearing-impaired people also report feelings of restricted social participation during breaks, that their career advancement was affected by the hearing loss, and that management had a negative perception of workers with occupational hearing loss.

In the study by Laroche, Garcia and Barette (2000), some individual factors were also mentioned as barriers. The nature of the hearing loss and its symptoms, e.g. physical fatigue, was one such barrier, and some other psychological factors that were mentioned included perception of self, lack of self-esteem, reluctance to express needs and unwillingness to disclose. The latter barriers were mentioned only by the audiologists; the hearing-impaired people themselves pointed to feelings of isolation and the need to hide their impairment (p. 80). The fact that they mentioned that they sometimes had to hide their impairment indicates problems in the attitudes among peers. This was investigated by Hétu, Getty and Waridel (1994) and Hétu et al. (1994), who found that, although there was a generally favourable attitude towards hearing-impaired co-workers, there was a 'a strong social desirability bias' (Hétu, Getty and Waridel, 1994, p. 299).

The fact that hard-of-hearing people face problems in their working life is supported by a substantial body of research. It is well documented in two recent large studies from Sweden and Denmark (Danermark and Coniavitis Gellerstedt, 2003, 2004b; Clausen, 2003). Both these studies showed that the psychosocial environment is more demanding for hard-of-hearing people than for normally hearing people. Danermark and Coniaivits Gellerstedt found that the most important difference between the study group and the control group was the lower degree of control over the work (see also Backenroth et al., 2003). They emphasized that this is an important factor in relation to health and emotional status. According to Karasek and Theorell's (1990) demand–control model, an imbalance between demand and control of the work is associated with negative health outcomes. Danermark and Coniavitis Gellerstedt found that among those hard-of-hearing workers who had high demand and low control (so-called high-stress work) the prevalence of problems with their neck, back, sleeping, stomach and headache was much higher than among those with less stressful work situations. They were also more irritated, dissatisfied, inefficient, tired, tense or frustrated, and had concentration problems and a feeling of not being involved.

Although it seems that a substantial proportion of hearing-impaired people are excluded from the labour market by forced early retirement or long-term sick leave, we have not found any study focusing on this group. This is a major shortcoming in the literature, since it is most likely that the increasing number of slimmed-down organizations, focusing on flexibility and communication skills, will exacerbate the problem of marginalization in terms of exclusion from the labour market.

Economic life (d860–879)

One aspect of the ICF's 'major life areas' is economic life. Not much research has been done in this field. Among the few studies is one by Clarcq and Walter (undated). They investigated the return of individual and societal investments in higher education among deaf people and hard-of-hearing people. Although the model is not comprehensive, in terms of either the costs or the returns, the results show that the return was significant from both an individual and a societal perspective. After 25 years of work, deaf and hard-of-hearing graduates with a bachelor's degree earned on average $8986 per year more than deaf or hard-of-hearing people with only a high-school diploma. The latter were also three times as likely to be receiving social income support as the former.

Mowry (1988) concluded that the financial resources of both hard-of-hearing people and deaf people were considerably lower than among comparable employees. But there is an important difference between the groups among the unemployed. Hard-of-hearing people were very poor, but unemployed deaf people were not. They received (from Social Security Disability payments, etc.) more than twice as much as their hard-of-hearing fellows (average income was more than the employed hard-of-hearing people and about equal to employed deaf people). The result must be interpreted with caution because of the socio-economic bias (degree of 'welfare state' provision) and the transformation of the labour market over the past 15 years.

Environmental factors

Legal systems (e550)

An important aspect of social and civic life is whether deaf or hard-of-hearing people are over-represented in the prison population. However, there are few studies focusing on this issue. In a review of the literature Vernon and

Greenberg (1999) concluded that the prevalence of deaf and hard-of-hearing inmates in correctional facilities is – according to conservative estimates – at least double the proportion found in the general population (10-15% compared to 5% in the general population). They also address the broader question of the relationship between deafness or hearing loss and violence. They point to three factors that might contribute to this state of affairs: 'educational, communicative, and vocational limitations associated with hearing loss; the increased rate of brain damage in this population; and the higher rate of learning disabilities among the hearing-impaired' (pp. 263-264). It is notable that the authors point out three individualistic factors – attributes within the individuals. From our ICF perspective there are many other important factors to highlight: environmental factors such as the educational system, social support and supported employment.

Vernon and Rich (1997) focused on another aspect of violence and criminal behaviour, paedophilia. In a descriptive study of 22 cases (20 male and 2 female deaf paedophiles) the authors found that most of them had a history of being sexually abused as children, had experienced mental disorders and had a criminal record.

In a study of inmates in Canadian penitentiaries, Dahl (1994) found that hard-of-hearing inmates were, to a large extent, over-represented among the prisoners. These inmates felt that they were not properly understood by either their peers or the prison staff and they felt they were discriminated against by the staff. She concluded that the behaviour of hard-of-hearing people was, in general, interpreted in negative terms.

Access to information (e5601)

One important aspect of civil life is having access to information, including the ability to watch television programmes. Without subtitles it is very difficult for some hard-of-hearing people to understand programmes such as news or debates. According to Sancho-Aldridge and Davis (1993), hard-of-hearing viewers report much greater difficulties watching programmes than viewers with no hearing problems. The problems are strongly correlated with age. For instance, in the hearing loss age group 18-50 about 24% reported moderate viewing difficulties compared to about 41% for the age group 51-80. The corresponding figures for people with no hearing problems were about 3% in both age groups.

Personal contextual factors

In this section we deal with psychiatric disorders, coping styles, overall behaviour pattern and character style, and individual psychological assets (see Table 5.1).

Early-onset deafness

Emotions

Emotional effects are one personal factor that is repeatedly mentioned in the literature; they include psychological effects such as paranoia, depression and other personality characteristics.

There are studies that report a higher prevalence of paranoia and depression among deaf people but, in a review of a number of reports dealing with this type of maladjustment, Meadow-Orlans (1985) points out that the results are contradictory. This is also underlined by Erdman and Demorest (1998) and by Schirmer (2001) who emphasized that the results are, at best, equivocal. They stress that this is not only the case for paranoia and depression.

However, it is important to address two different perspectives on development and functioning of people with early-onset deafness. One, the 'deviance model', focuses on the assumed consequences of deafness in terms of negative differences from hearing people. Studies from the 1930s to the 1970s mainly addressed the question of atypical behaviour. Many of the studies from this period are either anecdotal or have a flawed research design. The other perspective regards the socio-emotional development as basically the same for deaf and for hearing people and 'emphasizes the conditions necessary for the development of a healthy, whole, well-integrated person' (Moores, 1996). Over recent decades the latter perspective has become more and more influential and recent studies are both consistent with findings in other areas of disability research and unequivocal regarding the question of psychosocial maladjustment among those with early-onset deafness, although there are some studies that report a greater occurrence of different psychosocial problems among deaf people. Galán et al. (2000) found significant differences in hypochondria, hysteria, paranoia, psychasthenia and schizophrenia between pre- and postlingually deaf people on the one hand and hearing subjects on the other. Leigh, Robins and Welkowits (1990) and Danermark, Sjöström and Borg (1997) found significantly higher levels of mild depression among deaf people. These findings indicate that deafness is a risk factor, but the ambiguous findings show that it is a very complex multifactorial phenomenon and that there are some factors that might affect deaf people more than hearing people in relation to emotional and behavioural problems (Schirmer, 2001).

Identity among congenitally deaf people has been the subject of many studies and there is a considerable body of literature on this issue. However, since the research focuses on the early development of congenitally deaf people, it has been dealt with in the previous chapter. In the following section of this chapter we deal with the identity issue related to late-onset hearing impairment.

Late-onset deafness

Emotions

Relatively few studies (for an overview see Rutman, 1989; Rothschild and Kampfe, 1998) have investigated the emotional consequences of postlingual profound hearing loss. People in this group have the experience of hearing and speech and were brought up in an oral world. At the time of onset, they rarely have any experience or knowledge of Deafness and Deaf culture. Their identity is founded in the ability to hear, and they are confronted with a loss of their self-image (David and Trehub, 1989). Although many congenitally deaf people view their deafness in terms of differences and belonging to a language minority group, the acquired group view their deafness as a deficit. It is surprising that, compared with congenitally deaf people, this group has not been the focus of many well-controlled empirical studies even though they account for approximately 78% of all deaf people in the USA (Rothschild and Kampfe, 1998; Aguayo and Coady, 2001). Although we do not know the overall proportion in EU countries, they constitute a very large group, about three-quarters of those with severe hearing loss (70 dB or greater in the better ear).

The Past President of the Association of Late-Deafened Adults, Marylyn Howe, describes the psychosocial ramifications for this group of people (Howe, 1993). On the basis of reports from Jackson (1982), Nowell (1985) and Reiter (1990), Howe described this group as being viewed as 'aloof, withdrawn, depressed, passive, and/or over-reactive.' (p. 10). A basic problem is that they seldom develop any new mode of communication and, hence, late onset of deafness strikes at the very core of the human being where communication is the foundation and will affect all interpersonal interactions. Howe's characterization of the experiences of adventitious deafness received much support in the literature. Such individuals are at a greater risk of psychiatric disorders than congenitally deaf people and they are more likely to experience significant psychological and social problems (Rutman, 1989). Among the emotional consequences are mood disorders such as denial, anger, guilt, embarrassment, shame, frustration, helplessness, feelings of emptiness and acceptance (see e.g. David and Trehub, 1989; Jones and White, 1990; Kampfe, 1990; Kampfe and Smith, 1997; Kerr and Cowie, 1997). Both Luey (1980) and Kyle, Jones and Wood (1985) have developed a model of phases of acquired deafness, beginning with denial and ending with acceptance. It is postulated that it is very difficult for these deaf people to reach the final stage of acceptance, because it requires 'constant adjustment and readjustment to new roles, relationships, jobs, activities, and to a world of unending silence' (Rutman, 1989, p. 307). Using the Nottingham Health Profile, measuring health-related quality of life among people with severe–profound hearing impairment (sensorineural hearing loss in the better ear of > 70 dB at a frequency of 1.0 kHz), Ringdahl and Grimby (2000; see also Grimby and Ringdahl, 2000) found that these individuals reported a lower health-related quality of life than a normally hearing reference population. Among the factors that were reported as being worse than in the normally hearing group were social isolation, emotional reactions and lack of energy. The authors noted that women are more vulnerable than men, and concluded that 'the profoundly hearing-impaired persons seem to constitute a risk group for worse psychosocial adjustment and need greater attention and support' (p. 266).

However, it is very important to stress that responses to late-onset deafness are highly variable. Some people accept the loss without major difficulty, but some experience severe emotional problems. From the existing literature it is difficult to estimate the extent of the emotional trauma resulting from late-onset deafness, but many studies indicate that the emotional consequences are obvious. For instance, Aguayo and Coady (2001) reported that all eight respondents in the in-depth interviews experienced deep anxiety, grief and mourning. Thomas and Herbst (1980) are critical of much of the research published before 1980 and stress that many of the results are contradictory. In their own study they found no straightforward relationship between severity of hearing loss and psychological disturbance. However, they found that, for a small subsample of 23 respondents who had severe hearing loss coupled with poor speech discrimination ability, this was associated with psychological disturbances (Thomas, 1981). It is also important to stress that, as for congenitally deaf people, adventitious deafness seems not to be associated with psychotic illness (Rutman, 1989). In their review of the literature on this subject, Jones and White (1990) found that the claim that hearing loss is aetiologically related to mental illness – a claim that was common between 1960 and 1980 – has not been supported by more recent studies. The results are contradictory, and the quality of some of the studies does not permit a definitive conclusion.

There seems to be overwhelming support for the view that late-onset deafness is associated with emotional stress such as depression, but there is one study that does not confirm this (Galán et al., 2000). Galán and his colleagues found that depression (using an abbreviated version of the Minnesota Multiple Personality Inventory [MMPI]) was not significantly correlated with deafness. However, their conclusion is further developed and they state that unemployed postlingually deaf people have higher scores for depression, among other variables. We will return to this finding when dealing with consequences for employment.

While most researchers focus on problems and negative consequences, Hallberg, Påsse and Ringdahl (2000) chose to focus on health-promoting aspects, e.g. successful coping with activity limitations. Based on Antonowsky's (1987) salutogentic perspective, they investigated how severely hard-of-hearing people (> 70 dB hearing loss at 1 kHz in the better ear) coped with communication hindrance in everyday life. A successful coping strategy seemed to be to direct and manage those in the close environment, e.g. teaching people how to behave in order to adjust to the wishes and needs of the hearing-impaired individual.

People with unilateral sudden sensorineural hearing loss form a special subgroup. We have found only a few studies focusing on this group. Among the consequences Chiossoine-Kerdel et al. (2001) found that this group reported hearing handicap and tinnitus handicap. Another study indicated some 'communication and psychosocial problems' but we have very limited knowledge of the consequences for this group of hearing-impaired people.

Identity

As touched on above, late-onset deafness has severe effects on identity. Besides the loss of an identity, people with late-onset deafness are in a sense homeless since they do not belong either to the hearing world or to the deaf community – they are 'between worlds' (Luey, 1980). A sense of isolation is therefore very common: even in the family, the feeling of isolation is often profound. To be in-between is to be marginalized. This is a very serious state since, as Rutman writes (1989, p. 309), referring to Sussman (1965), 'a "marginal" person begins to adjust only when he or she can gain a sense of identity with one world of another'. Although the literature does not give much information as to whether members of this group of deaf people strive to belong to the deaf community or the hearing world, Rutman (1989) suggests that it is more common for them to identify with the hearing world. There are many reasons for this, including lack of communication skills, ignorance of the Deaf community, and attitudes among both the groups of deaf and the surrounding environment (David and Trehub, 1989).

Hard-of-hearing

Consequences related to the time for onset for hard-of-hearing people have been the subject of some studies. The overall result is that there are only minor differences between early onset or late onset in terms of effects (e.g. Parving and Christensen, 1993; Danermark and Coniavitis Gellersted, 2003). In the following section we will not therefore discuss the consequences for these two groups separately.

There are a number of individual effects for hard-of-hearing people. One category of effects is closely related to the impairment itself. Hétu, Getty and

Quoc (1995) describe six individual effects of hearing impairment and the nature of the hearing loss (pp. 496–497):

- Loss of hearing sensitivity, i.e. a sound below the threshold of detection is not perceived.
- Compressed loudness function, which means that the range between inaudibility and clear audibility is sometimes very small.
- Loss of frequency resolution. When there are competing sounds it is very difficult for a hearing-impaired person to 'select' the sound they want to listen to.
- Loss of temporal resolution – the ability to recognize gaps in an ongoing sound.
- Loss of spatial resolution is a well-documented consequence. It is difficult to recognize where the sound is coming from, which affects the possibility of orienting one's attention towards its source.
- Persistence of annoying tinnitus. This is a common phenomenon among hard-of-hearing people and can result in problems with rest and sleep.

Identity

There is an important difference between hard-of-hearing identity and Deaf culture. The latter has a strong social and cultural dimension. To be Deaf is to have a cultural group membership. This is not the case for hard-of-hearing people. Laszlo (1994) and Getty and Hétu (1994) point out that hard-of-hearing people are heterogeneous in terms of social experiences, and the basis for developing common shared values and norms is absent.

However, there has been a discussion as to whether or not there is a hard-of-hearing identity. Ford (1992) argued that there is such an identity. One of his arguments is the increasing establishment of hard-of-hearing organizations, and his interpretation is that there is a specific hard-of-hearing group identity, in between the hearing and the Deaf worlds. On the other hand, Danermark and Coniavitis Gellerstedt (2004a, 2004b) emphasized that hard-of-hearing people do not have a unifying group identity. People with hearing loss are not really members of a group with a specific, commonly felt cultural identity. Rather, it is other people who impose a stereotyped identity, assigning characteristics such as *slow, tiresome, less intelligent* to people with hearing loss. This does not, of course, mean that people with hearing loss do not share experiences and claims that are rooted in their hearing impairment. People with hearing loss frequently experience institutionalized patterns that designate them as less than full members of society and prevent them from participating as peers in social life. Examples of such institutionalized patterns are lack of FM radio systems or loop systems in lecture halls and theatres, or high levels of noise in workplaces, i.e. circumstances that generate claims for redistribution of material resources and so have financial implications. People with hearing impairment thus hardly require recognition of a group-specific *identity*. Laszlo is also sceptical about the arguments for a specific hard-of-hearing identity and community, and concludes 'There is certainly no convincing evidence that hard-of-hearing people prefer the hard-of-hearing community in any cultural sense' (1994, p. 252). This statement was further underlined by Getty and Hétu (1994), who did not find any empirical support for a hard-of-hearing culture of workers with hearing loss.

Mental health and emotions

Some studies report a high prevalence of negative emotions such as frustration, stress, anger and resentment. Regarding mental health, the results are conflicting, except for mild depression. Some studies indicate abnormal personality, some do not. The same is true for paranoia (for an overview see Jones and White, 1990). Hétu, Lalonde and Getty (1987) also point to a negative self-image as an important consequence. Danermark and Coniavitis Gellerstedt (2003) (see below) reported a number of health and emotional factors among hard-of-hearing people. Loneliness and a sense of isolation – in the workplace, in the family and in other social settings – are very frequently reported and were discussed under 'Family' and 'Work and career', respectively.

Although many studies mention emotional problems among hard-of-hearing people, only a few focus or elaborate on the issue. Many studies addressing this issue do not separate deaf and hard-of-hearing in their analyses. This is the case for some of the studies referred to at the beginning of this chapter and, as a result, we do not know if the over-representation concerns deaf or hard-of-hearing people or if both groups are affected.

Fatigue

One of the most noticeable effects of hearing impairment is fatigue or lack of energy. Both physical and mental tiredness have been documented in the literature (e.g. Antonson, 1998; Ringdal and Grimby, 2000; Backenroth et al., 2003; Danermark and Coniavitis Gellerstedt, 2004b). In his study of hearing-impaired students, Antonson identified three types of fatigue, one that was the 'same for everybody', one that was a result of the effort of listening and a third type that was a consequence of a specific activity, for instance the absence of a good learning method or, more generally speaking, good coping strategies. Tiredness could also be a result of making oneself understood (Oyer and Oyer, 1979). Tiredness seems to be a common problem, especially for working hearing-impaired people (Hétu et al., 1988). Danermark and Coniavitis Gellerstedt (2004b) report a significantly higher degree of problems with sleep among hearing-impaired people compared with a normally hearing reference population. For instance, 46% of hearing-impaired women had problems with sleep at least once a week compared to 22% of a reference population. Problems with sleep were very closely correlated with tiredness (χ^2 = 46. 6, d.f. = 4, p = 0.000). In the qualitative part of their analysis they found that one reason for this was that, after a full day at work, the hearing-impaired people had to take a nap and this made it more difficult to get to sleep later (see also Hétu, Lalonde and Getty, 1987). Another reason for problems with sleep was tinnitus. Nervousness and other common types of stressful feelings are also a source of tiredness.

Another group of people with hearing impairment is those with unilateral hearing loss. There are two subgroups: early and late onset. There is no evidence in the literature that the first group is subject to consequences related to the hearing loss (see Colletti et al., 1988). However, in the group of late onset of unilateral hearing loss, Chiossoine-Kerdel et al. (2000) reported that, for those with sudden hearing loss, 57% reported tinnitus handicap and 86% reported hearing handicap.

The last group of people with hearing difficulties to be considered in this overview are those with the King–Kopetzky syndrome (KKS), sometimes labelled obscure auditory dysfunction. People suffering from this syndrome are characterized by hearing difficulties in background noise, despite normal audiograms. Most of the literature in this field deals with the clinical characterization of this group, since knowledge of the aetiology is very limited. It has been suggested that it is either auditory or psychological or a combination of the two (Saunders and Haggard, 1989) and that it could have a genetic cause since there is an over-representation of a family history of hearing problems among those with KKS (Stephens and Zhao, 2000). Not much has been reported in terms of psychosocial consequences, but the findings indicate that the problems are very much like those reported by hard-of-hearing people with auditory measurable limitations, such as loneliness, anxiety and mild depression (King and Stephens, 1992). Further, Stephens and Zhao (2000) provided some evidence suggesting that men with this condition and a family history showed higher levels of anxiety and obsessionality than those without such a family history.

Conclusions

What conclusions can be drawn from this overview? Although we have not been able to trace all the literature reporting findings on consequences of hearing impairment in the working-age population, we are confident that we have a sufficient body of research reports to allow us to draw some valid conclusions.

However, given the aim of this book it is important to note first and foremost that the literature does not give us any clue regarding different psychosocial impact of hearing impairment in adults with genetic and non-genetic aetiologies. Some studies give a hint that there might be some differences, but these differences have not been sufficiently demonstrated scientifically. The main differences that are shown in the literature are between prelingual and postlingual hearing impairment.

Most of the studies mentioned in this chapter are quantitative. The number of subjects varies, but in most studies they do not exceed 100 and only a few studies have a population of more than 200 subjects. The small number of subjects, in combination with statistical quantitative methods that very often require specific conditions for the analysis that are sometimes not fulfilled, makes the conclusions very shaky. Furthermore, although we have found some follow-up studies, only one 'real' longitudinal study has been found, and no study applying a lifetime design. This is an important short-coming since, as we have described, hearing impairment and hearing loss are processes, not fixed and stable conditions. That means there is a great need for analyses that can catch the dynamic aspects of the issue and we conclude that such analyses are very few. Unfortunately, the longitudinal study we mentioned had a drop-out rate of 50%. Most longitudinal studies have signifi-cant drop-outs, but the problem with drop-outs was not addressed in this paper and hence there was no discussion of its impact on the conclusions. It is plausible to assume that the unwillingness to participate is correlated with the issue under investigation – job or career. Those who had been less successful might be less willing to admit this, and more reluctant to partici-pate. We do not know if this was the case, but if it were so the results would be seriously flawed.

Who are the hearing-impaired people whom we know about? Almost every study reported here uses clinic populations. With a few exceptions, such as prisoners or paedophiles, we do not have much psychosocial data on hearing-impaired people who are not patients. There are indications that many hearing-impaired people are not registered at any clinic, and that this group is significantly younger (Danermark and Coniavitis Gellerstedt, 2003).

Another weakness is that many studies do not include any reference data (e.g. matched reference group, general population) which makes it difficult to assess the findings in terms of 'over-representation'. The question of refer-ence group is not a simple one. For instance, studies reporting more stress among hard-of-hearing people might use a matched control group of normally hearing people. However, a control group consisting of people who have experienced the loss of a breast after cancer surgery, or loss of a partner, might not show a higher level of stress than hearing-impaired people. It might be a normal reaction to a loss of something that is an integrated part of one's identity or everyday life. Such findings would throw new light on the relationship between hearing loss and emotional reactions.

The final methodological issue is the information that is provided about the subjects. Although the research is conducted by scholars who are familiar with the topic, surprisingly few collect or present sufficient data about, for example, time of onset and degree of hearing loss. As we will explain, such variables are important for conclusions about the consequences of hearing impairment.

In short, from a methodological perspective, the quality and definition of hearing impairment, sample characteristics, methodologies and outcome measures differ and make comparisons between studies difficult.

Descriptive conclusions relate to the consequences of hearing loss – the central theme of this book. Given the shortcomings described above, there are some findings that are well documented and seem very robust. As mentioned in the introduction to this chapter, the term 'consequences of hearing impairment. . . ' implies a causal relationship – if A then B – but very few studies have been designed to provide us with such a causal conclusion. Most often they end up with statistical correlations that are at best supported by some theoretical arguments, but mostly the causality seems to be implicitly assumed. This is further underlined in WHO's presentation of the ICF classification framework (2001):

> To infer a limitation in capacity from one or more impairments, or a restriction of performance from one or more limitations, may often seem reasonable. It is important, however, to collect data on these constructs independently and thereafter explore associations and causal links between them (p. 19).

Statements of causal links have to be theoretically justified and, since quantitative research often lacks theoretical elaboration, many of the reported correlations between hearing impairment and the investigated psychosocial variables cannot be taken to be causally related without further investigations. As we shall see, there are tendencies to develop theories about hearing impairment and different types of outcomes but they are seldom brought to the fore in the quantitative studies we have found.

Another feature of this type of research is that it seldom includes structural conditions, but mostly focuses on the individual. This shortcoming is to some extent 'embedded' in the quantitative approach and research design. It is very difficult to perform traditional statistical analyses including variables at different levels (biological, psychological, socio-economic and cultural).

In this overview we have found some general and common features in terms of psychosocial effects of being hearing-impaired. For some hearing-impaired people there are negative emotional consequences; for others there seem to be no significant consequences. People with late-onset deafness seem to be an especially high-risk group. This group also seems to have identity problems. Both deaf and hard-of-hearing people report communication problems, but of a different character. Deaf people have no problem when the communication partner uses sign language, but hard-of-hearing people always seem to have problems in non-ideal communication environments. For hard-of-hearing people, these communication problems tend to have effects on their social life, in some cases severe. In their working life, many hearing-impaired people are subject to different forms of lack of recognition, such as less career advancement than normally hearing peers. They experience isolation and less respect from their hearing associates. There are some indications that unemployment is more common among hearing-impaired people than among the normally hearing. However, this is not always the case, e.g. in Sweden. We have little knowledge about hearing impairment and unemployment.

The issue of gender has been addressed in only very few studies. Deaf and hard-of-hearing people are treated as a unisex group. There are studies indicating that there is a difference between men and women regarding psychosocial effects (e.g. Hétu, Jones and Getty, 1993; Hallberg and Jansson, 1996; Danermark and Coniavitis Gellerstedt, 2003) and there are studies indicating that there are no significant differences (e.g. Clausen, 2003). There is a need for further research from a gender perspective.

Qualitative studies are often designed to search for fundamental characteristics of a particular phenomenon. For instance, when investigating communication problems between deaf and hearing people, Foster (1998) identified three categories of communication problems (see above). Another example is Hallberg and Carlsson (1991) who identified two categories of coping strategies for dealing with demanding auditory situations in everyday life: controlling the social scene or avoiding it. These categories are deduced from empirical observations. The researchers use different strategies to create the categories. For instance, Foster articulated a theory as point of departure whereas Hallberg and Carlsson were more inductive in the development of categories. Although all categorization is underpinned by theory and all observations are theory-laden, this is often not made explicit and it is difficult to see to what extent it has guided the researcher in the analysis. In addition, there are some studies claiming to use qualitative methods which only report what the respondents say without any analysis of the text.

There are fewer qualitative studies than quantitative ones. The results from these studies confirm many of the findings in the qualitative studies. The qualitative studies we have reported here focus mainly on communication and/or emotional aspects of hearing impairment in different settings (mainly education and working life). There are only a few qualitative studies that include deaf people. A reason for this could be the need to use sign language. Although these studies do not tell us how common psychosocial effects are and how they statistically correlate with different characteristics of the subject and the environment, they do give us good knowledge about different types of (coping) behaviour and a better understanding of what it means to be hearing-impaired.

Are the correlations between hearing impairment and associated variables revealed in this review causal in nature, and do the qualitative studies help us to better understand the processes in causal terms? There are some attempts in the literature to theorize the issue. Goffman's (1967) elaboration of Mead's theory of symbolic interaction plays a vital role here. Stigmatization is the fundamental psychosocial process that explains many of the social findings. One could say that the theory of symbolic interaction and stigmatization dominates the theoretical discourse in relation to hard-of-hearing people. The theory of symbolic interaction applied to hard-of-hearing people has been elaborated by Hétu and his colleagues in a number of articles (see, for example, Hétu, 1996). By introducing Honneth's (1995) theory of social recognition and Fraser's (1995) theory of redistribution of resources, the issue has been further developed by Danermark and Coniavitis Gellerstedt (2003, 2004a,b). In relation to deafness, Emerton (e.g. 1992) presented a theoretical framework based on symbolic interaction in which he developed the concepts of 'marginality' and 'biculturalism'.

Another non-competing strand is a framework based mainly on the ecological approach of Gibson and Bronfenbrenner. This has been put forward by Foster, Noble and their colleagues (e.g. Noble, 1983; Foster and DeCaro, 1990; Foster, 1991).

Despite the critique presented here we strongly argue that the empirical findings presented and discussed in this chapter provide clear evidence of a theoretical understanding of the relationship between hearing impairment and many of the psychosocial consequences reported in the literature. Hearing impairment generates problems in verbal communication. This communication difficulty is the basic mechanism that in turn produces, alone or in conjunction with other mechanisms, emotional reactions, stigmatization, isolation, career problems, lack of social recognition and so forth. However, it is of the utmost importance to bear in mind that the outcome of the interplay between different mechanisms depends on individual characteristics (e.g. level of hearing loss, time of onset) and structural conditions (e.g. norms, values, legislation). That means that an important characteristic of this field of research is its multidisciplinarity nature (see Danermark, 2002). Biological, psychological and cultural processes all have effects on the consequences of hearing impairment. Therefore it is an important but difficult task to investigate these processes, trying to answer the question 'For *whom* will a hearing impairment result in *what* under *which circumstances?*'. In order to achieve a better understanding of these processes we need theoretically informed multidisciplinary research, including longitudinal studies, drawing samples that allow us to make more specific conclusions in terms of *who*, *what* and *which* than we have so far been able to do.

To be able to address the question of psychosocial consequences of *genetic* hearing impairment, first there is a great need for studies that include an aetiological perspective, e.g. family history. Secondly, there is also a general need for theoretically well-informed, longitudinal and multidisciplinary studies, which include a gender perspective, in more or less all the fields that have been discussed in this chapter.

References

Aguayo MO, Coady NF (2001) The experience of deafened adults: implications for rehabilitative services. Health and Social Work 26: 269–276.

Allen TE (1986) Patterns of academic achievement among hearing-impaired students: 1975 and 1983. In: Schildroth AN, Karchmer MA (eds) Deaf Children in America. College-Hill Press, San Diego, pp. 161–206.

Antonowsky A (1987) Unravelling the Mystery of Health: how people manage stress and stay well. Jossey-Bass, San Francisco, CA.

Antonson S (1998) Hörselskadade i högskolestudier. Möjligheter och hinder (Diss. No. 59). Linköpings Universitet, Linköping, Sweden.

Backenroth G (1995) Deaf people's perception of social interaction in working life. International Journal of Rehabilitation Research 18: 76–81.

Backenroth GAM, Ohsako P, Wennberg AF, Klinteberg B (2003) Personality and work life: a comparison between hearing impaired persons and a normal hearing population. Social Behaviour and Personality 31: 191–204.

Caisse R, Rockwell E (1993) A videotape analysis procedure for assessing conversational fluency in hearing-impaired adults. Ear and Hearing 14: 202–209.

Calderon R, Greenberg MT (1999) Stress and coping in hearing mothers of children with hearing loss: factors affecting mother and child adjustment. American Annals of the Deaf 144: 7–18.

Carlsson P-I, Danermark B, Borg E (2004) Marital status and number of children born among deaf people in Sweden. The impact of the social environment in terms of Deaf community, American Annals of the Deaf.

Chiossoine-Kerdel J, Baguley D, Stoddart R, Moffat D (2000) An investigation of the audiologic handicap associated with unilateral sudden sensorineural hearing loss. American Journal of Otology 21: 645–651.

Clarcq JR, Walter GG (undated) Assessing the Benefits of Postsecondary Education. National Technical Institution for the Deaf, Rochester, NY.

Clausen T (2003) Når hørelsen svigter [When Hearing Flinches]. 03:01. Socialforskningsinstituttet, Copenhagen.

Colletti V, Fiorino F, Carner M, Rizzi R (1988) Investigation of the long-term effects of unilateral hearing loss in adults. British Journal of Audiology 22: 113–118.

Cowie RID, Stewart P (1987) Acquired deafness and the family: a problem for psychologists. Irish Journal of Psychology viii: 138–154.

Dahl M (1994) Hard-of-hearing inmates in penitentiaries. Journal of Speech Language Pathology and Audiology 18: 271–277.

Danermark B (2002) Interdisciplinary research and critical realism. The example of disability research. Journal of Critical Realism 5: 56–64.

Danermark B, Coniavitis Gellerstedt L (2003) Att höra till – om hörselskadades psykosociala arbetsmiljö [Belonging – On Psychosocial Working Conditions of People with Hearing Impairment]. Örebro Universitet, Örebro, Sweden.

Danermark B, Coniavitis Gellerstedt L (2004a) Social justice: redistribution and recognition – a non-reductionist perspective on disability. Disability and Society 19: 339–353.

Danermark B, Coniavitis Gellerstedt L (2004b) Hearing impairment, psychosocial work environment and health. International Journal of Audiology in press.

Danermark B, Sjöström L, Borg B (1997) Some characteristics of mainstreamed hard of hearing students in Swedish universities. American Annals of the Deaf 5: 359–364.

David M, Trehub SE (1989) Perspectives on deafened adults. American Annals of the Deaf 134: 200–204.

The Deaf Canadian Magazine (1981) Editorial. The Deaf Canadian Magazine (September issue).

DeCaro J, Mudgett-DeCaro P, Dowliby F (2001) Attitudes toward occupations for deaf youth in Sweden. American Annals of the Deaf 146: 51–59.

El-Khaime A (1993) Employment transitions and establishing careers by postsecondary alumni with hearing loss. Volta Review 95: 357–366.

Emerton G (1992) Marginality and Biculturalism: effects on the development of social identity of deaf people. Rochester Institute of Technology/NTID, Rochester, NY.

Erdman SA, Demorest ME (1998) Adjustment to hearing impairment II: audiological and demographic correlates. Journal of Speech, Language, and Hearing Research 41: 123–136.

Fisiloglu AG, Fisiloglu H (1996) Turkish families with deaf and hard of hearing children: a systems approach in assessing family functioning. American Annals of the Deaf 141: 231–235.

Ford J (1992) Hard of hearing people: Are we a community? Are we a culture? In: Congress Report of the 4th International Congress of Hard of Hearing People. MD Enterprises, Port Coquitlam, BC, pp. 66–68.

Foster S (1987) Employment experiences of deaf college graduates: an interview study. Journal of the Rehabilitation of the Deaf 21: 1–15.

Foster S (1991) An ecological model of social interaction between deaf and hearing students within a postsecondary educational setting. Disability, Handicap and Society 6: 181–201.

Foster S (1992) Accommodation of deaf college graduates in the workplace. In: Foster S, Walter G (ed.) Deaf Students in Post-secondary Education. Routledge, London, pp. 210–235.

Foster S (1998) Communication as social engagement: implications for interactions between deaf and hearing persons. Scandinavian Audiology, Supplementum 49: 116–124.

Foster S, DeCaro P (1990) Mainstreaming hearing-impaired students within a postsecondary educational setting: an ecological model of social interaction. Paper presented at the Annual Meeting of the American Educational Research Association in Boston, 18 April 1990, Boston, MA.

Foster S, MacLeod J (2003) Deaf people at work: assessment of communication among deaf and hearing persons in work settings. International Journal of Audiology 43 (suppl 1): 128–139.

Fraser N (1995) From redistribution to recognition? dilemmas of justice in a 'post-socialist' age. New Left Review 212(July/August): 68–93.

Gagné J-P, Wyllie K (1989) Relative effectiveness of three repair strategies on the visual identification of misperceived words. Ear and Hearing 10: 368–374.

Galán S, Sánchez D, Ramón D, Canizo A del, Fernandez-Roldán A (2000) Personality study in profoundly deaf adults. Review of Laryngology, Otology and Rhinology 121: 339–343.

Getty L, Hétu R (1994) Is there a culture of hard-of-hearing workers? Journal of Speech Language Pathology and Audiology 18: 267–270.

Glass L, Elliott H (1992) The professionals told me that it was, but that's not enough. SHHH Journal: 26–28.

Goffman E (1967) Interaction Ritual – essays on face-to-face behavior. Anchor Books, New York.

Grimby A, Ringdahl A (2000) Does having a job improve the quality of life among post-lingually deafened Swedish adults with severe-profound hearing impairment? British Journal of Audiology 34: 187–195.

Hallberg L (1999) Hearing impairment, coping and consequences on family life. Journal of the Academy of Rehabilitative Audiology 32: 45–59.

Hallberg L, Barrenäs ML (1993) Living with a male with noise-induced hearing loss. Experiences from the perspectives of spouses. British Journal of Audiology 27: 255–261.

Hallberg L, Carlsson S (1991) A qualitative study of strategies for managing a hearing impairment. British Journal of Audiology 25: 201–211.

Hallberg L, Jansson G (1996) Women with noise-induced hearing loss: an invisible group? British Journal of Audiology 30: 340–345.

Hallberg LR, Påsse U, Ringdahl A (2000) Coping with post-lingual severe-profound hearing impairment: a grounded theory study. British Journal of Audiology 34: 1–9.

Hétu R (1996) The stigma attached to hearing impairment. Scandinavian Audiology 25: (suppl 43) 12–24.

Hétu R, Getty L, Quoc H (1995) Impact of occupational hearing loss in the lives of workers. Occupational Medicine 10: 495–512.

Hétu R, Getty L, Waridel S (1994) Attitudes towards co-workers affected by occupational hearing loss II: focus group interviews. British Journal of Audiology 28: 313–325.

Hétu R, Jones L, Getty L (1993) The impact of acquired hearing impairment on intimate relationships: implications for rehabilitation. Audiology 32: 363–81.

Hétu R, Lalonde M, Getty L (1987) Psychosocial disadvantages associated with occupational hearing loss as experienced in the family. Audiology 26: 141–152.

Hétu R, Riverin L, Lalande N, Getty L, St-Cyr C (1988) Qualitative analysis of the handicap associated with occupation hearing loss. British Journal of Audiology 22: 251–264.

Hétu R, Getty L, Beaudry J, Philibert L (1994) Attitudes towards co-workers affected by occupational hearing loss I: questionnaire development and inquiry. British Journal of Audiology 28: 299–311.

Holmes SA (1994) In 4 years, disabilities act hasn't improved jobs rate. New York Times, 23 October, p. 22.

Honneth A (1995) The Struggle for Recognition. The grammar of social conflict. Polity Press, Cambridge.

Howe M (1993) Meeting the needs of late-deafened adults. American Rehabilitation (Winter issue).

Huttunen K, Sorri M, Väyryen M et al. (1999) Educational outcome and employment of Finns with prelingual genetic vs non-genetic hearing impairment – a 15 year follow up. European Work Group on Genetics of Hearing Impairment Infoletter 6: 36–37.

Jackson P (1982) The psychological and economic profile of the hearing-impaired adult. In: Hull R (ed.) Rehabilitative audiology. Grune & Stratton, New York, pp. 27–33.

Jones L, Kyle J, Wood P (1987) Words Apart: losing your hearing as an adult. Tavistock Press, London.

Jones E, White A (1990) Mental health and acquired hearing impairment: a review. British Journal of Audiology 24: 3–9.

Järvelin MR, Mäki-Torkko E, Sorri M, Rantakallio PT (1997) Effect of hearing impairment on educational outcomes and employment up to the age of 25 years in northern Finland. British Journal of Audiology 31: 165–175.

Kampfe C (1990) Communication with persons who are deaf: Some practical suggestions for rehabilitation specialists. Journal of Rehabilitation 56: 41–45.

Kampfe C, Smith M (1997) Intrapersonal aspects of hearing loss in persons who are older. Journal of Rehabilitation 64: 24–29.

Karasek R, Theorell T (1990) Healthy Work. Stress, productivity, and the reconstruction of working life. Basic Books, New York.

Kerr PC, Cowie RID (1997) Acquired deafness. A multi-dimensional experience. British Journal of Audiology 31: 177–188.

King K, Stephens D (1992) Auditory and psychological factors in 'Auditory Disability with Normal Hearing'. Scandinavian Audiology 21: 109–114.

Koester LS, Meadow-Orlans KP (1999) Responses to interactive stress: Infants who are deaf or hearing. American Annals of the Deaf 144: 395–403.

Kyle J (1985) Deaf people: assessing the community or the handicap. Bulletin of the British Psychological Society 38: 137–141.

Kyle J, Wood J (1987) Adjustment to acquired deafness. British Association of Deafened People, London.

Kyle JG, Jones LG, Wood PL (1985) Adjustment to acquired hearing loss: A working model. In: Orlans H (ed.) Adjustment of Adult Hearing Loss. Taylor & Francis, London, pp. 119–138.

Lampropouplou V, Konstantareas M (1998) Child involvement and stress in Greek mothers of deaf children. American Annals of the Deaf 143: 296–30.

Laroche C, Garcia LJ, Barette J (2000) Perceptions by persons with hearing impairment, audiologists, and employers of the obstacles to work integration. Journal of the Academy of Rehabilitative Audiology 33: 63–90.

Laszlo C (1994) Is there a hard-of-hearing identity? Journal of Speech, Language Pathology and Audiology 18: 248–252.

Leigh IW, Robins CJ, Welkowits J (1990) Impact of communication on depressive vulnerability in deaf individuals. Journal of the American Deafness and Rehabilitation Association 23: 68–73.

Luey HS (1980) Between worlds: the problem of deafened adults. Social Work in Health Care 5: 253–265.

Mapp I, Hudson R (1997) Stress and coping among African American and Hispanic parents of deaf children. American Annals of the Deaf 142: 48–56.

Meadow-Orlans K (1985) Social and psychological effects of hearing loss in adulthood: a literature review. In: Orlans H (ed.) Adjustment of Adult Hearing Loss. Taylor & Francis, London.

Middleton A (1999) Attitudes of deaf and hearing individuals towards issues surrounding genetic testing for deafness. PhD Thesis, University of Leeds, UK.

Moores D (1996) Educating the Deaf. Psychology, principles, and practices. Houghton Mifflin, Boston, MA.

Moores D, Jatho J, Dunn C (2001) Families with deaf members: American Annals of the Deaf, 1996 to 2000. American Annals of the Deaf 146: 245–250.

Mowry RL (1988) Quality of life indicators for deaf and hard-of-hearing former VR clients. Journal of Rehabilitation for the Deaf 21(3): 1–7.

Mowry RL, Anderson GB (1993) Deaf adults tell their stories: perspectives on barriers to job. Volta Review 95: 367–377.

Noble W (1983) Hearing, hearing impairment and the audible world: a theoretical essay. Audiology 22: 325–338.

Nowell RC (1985) Psychology of hearing impaired. In: Katz J (ed.) Handbook of Clinical Audiology, 3rd edn. Williams & Wilkins, Baltimore, MD, pp. 776–786.

Oyer H, Oyer E (1979) Social consequences of hearing loss for the elderly. Allied Health and Behavioral Sciences 2: 133–136.

Parving A, Christensen B (1993) Training and employment in hearing-impaired subjects at 20–35 years of age. Scandinavian Audiology 22: 133–139.

Reiter RS (1990) Psychology of the hearing-impaired and hearing aid use: the art of dispensing. In: Sandlin R (ed.) Handbook of Hearing Aid Amplification, Volume II. College Hill Press, Boston, MA, pp. 1–30.

Ringdahl A, Grimby A (2000) Severe-profound hearing impairment and health related quality of life among post-lingual deafened Swedish adults. Scandinavian Audiology 29: 266–275.

Rothschild MA, Kampfe CM (1988) Issues associated with late onset deafness. Journal of the American Deafness and Rehabilitation Association 31(1): 1–16.

Rutman D (1989) The impact and experience of adventitious deafness. American Annals of the Deaf 134: 305–311.

Sancho-Aldridge J, Davis A (1993) The impact of hearing impairment on television viewing in the UK. British Journal of Audiology 27: 163–173.

Saunders G, Haggard M (1989) The clinical assessment of obscure auditory dysfunction – 1. Auditory and psychological factors. Ear and Hearing 10: 200–208.

Schein J (1982) The demography of deafness. In: Higgins P, Nash J (eds) The Deaf Community and Deaf Population. Gallaudet College, Washington, DC.

Scherich D, Mowry R (1997) Accomodations in the workplace for people who are hard of hearing: Perceptions of employees. Journal of the American Deafness and Rehabilitation Association 31(1): 31–43.

Schirmer B (2001) Psychological, Social, and Educational Dimensions of Deafness. Allyn & Bacon, Needham Heights, MA.

Schroedel JG (1976) Variables related to the attainment of occupational status among deaf adults. Doctoral dissertation, New York University. Dissertation Abstracts International 37(2).

Schroedel JG, Geyer PD (2001) Enhancing the careeer advancement of workers with hearing loss: results from a national follow-up survey. Journal of Applied Rehabilitation Counselling 32(3): 35–44.

Stephens D, France L, Lormore K (1995) Effects of hearing impairment on the patient's family and friends. Acta Otolaryngologica 115: 165–167.

Stephens D, Zhao F (2000) The role of family history in King Kopetzky syndrome (obscure auditory dysfunction). Acta Otolaryngologica 120: 197–200.

SOU (2001) Funktionshinder och välfärd [Disability and welfare]. SOU, Ministry of Social Affairs, Stockholm.

Thomas A (1981) Acquired deafness and mental health. British Journal of Medical Psychology 54: 219–229.

Thomas A, Herbst KG (1980) Social and psychological implications of acquired deafness for adults at employment age. British Journal of Audiology 14: 76–85.

Tye-Murray N, Witt S (1996) Conversational moves and conversational styles of adult cochlear-implant users. Journal of the Academy of Rehabilitative Audiology 29: 11–25.

Vernon G, Greenberg S (1999) Violence in deaf and hard-of-hearing people: A review of the literature. Aggression and Violent Behaviour 4: 259–272.

Vernon G, Rich S (1997) Pedophilia and deafness. American Annals of the Deaf 142: 300–311.

Welsh WA (1993) Factors influencing career mobility of deaf adults. Volta Review 95: 329–339.

Welsh WA, Walter G (1988) The effect of postsecondary education on the occupational attainments of deaf adults. Journal of the American Deafness and Rehabilitation Association 22(1): 14–22.

WHO (2001) International Classification of Functioning, Disability and Health – ICF. World Health Organization, Geneva, Switzerland.

Chapter 7

The psychosocial impact of hearing loss among elderly people: a review

Sophia Kramer

This chapter presents a review of articles published in the international literature on the psychosocial impact of hearing loss on elderly people. Exploration of the databases (for details see Chapter 4) yielded a large number of articles published in the last 20 years. The literature search found only a small number of studies dealing with the psychosocial impact of Deafness among elderly people. Also, no articles on the specific effects of genetic hearing impairment on the people affected and those around them were found.

A remarkable reflection of the present review is the wide variety of definitions ascribed to 'psychosocial health'. While some define it as *cognition*, others use terms such as *depression, neuroticism, loneliness, general wellbeing* or a combination of these. An even greater diversity is observed when the use of outcome measures – both generic and disease-specific – is considered (Table 7.1). The studies reviewed in this chapter mainly used self-report outcome measures and, while the vast majority of publications show adverse effects of hearing loss, conflicting evidence is found for some consequences. These contradictory outcomes are reported.

Learning and applying knowledge (d1); general tasks and demands (d2)

Integrating hearing loss into one's life requires constantly learning how to adapt to changes. It is a complex and dynamic process. It comprises developing new problem-solving skills, implementing new approaches, gaining information, changing and adding routines and the constant need to make adjustments. This is the conclusion of a qualitative study by Herth (1998). It reflects the experience and daily performance of many people with hearing loss aspiring to be involved in life. In addition, *handling stress* and *distraction*, subcategories under ICF d2, are well recognized and frequently experienced by individuals with auditory disability.

137

The aspects described above are elements of *cognitive functioning* which is, in many studies, considered as an essential domain of *psychosocial functioning*. Hearing loss, and particularly the process of integration and adjustment, depends greatly upon cognitive capacities. At the same time, a decline of cognitive functioning in older individuals with hearing impairment is a frequently observed phenomenon.

Using a variety of outcome measures to assess cognitive functioning (Table 7.1), a number of studies showed a significant association between hearing loss and cognitive decline, particularly among older adults.

In exploring the general role of auditory and visual functioning in cognitive ageing among 156 old and very old institutionalized individuals (70–103 years), Lindenberger and Baltes (1994) measured five different intellectual abilities: speed, reasoning, knowledge, memory and fluency. A strong connection between sensory decline and cognitive deterioration, including speed, was demonstrated.

In a large cross-sectional study of 1332 individuals aged 65–96 years, Cacciatore et al. (1999) found the Mini-Mental State Examination (MMSE) to be adversely related to hearing impairment, a greater loss implicating greater cognitive decline. Similar results were found in studies by Thomas et al. (1983), Naramura et al. (1999) and Bazargan, Baker and Bazargan (2001). Controlling for age, gender, educational level and processing speed, a mild-to-moderate hearing loss predicted lower verbal memory performance in a study by Van Boxtel et al. (2000).

The above studies evidently show a link between hearing loss and cognitive decline. However, it remains unknown whether cognitive deterioration causes hearing loss or, in turn, hearing loss causes cognitive decline. None of the above-mentioned studies could show causality. Besides this, there are a couple of studies which aimed to demonstrate an independent connection between hearing and cognitive capacities, but failed to do so. An example is the study of Carabellese et al. (1993) who examined the impact of hearing or visual impairments on the quality of life among a sample of 1191 elderly Italians, aged 70–75 years. The authors did not find an independent adverse effect of hearing loss on cognition. Only those with double sensory dysfunction were negatively affected.

It is worth noting here that the method used to test cognitive capacity may influence the outcome. Most of the tests described (e.g. MMSE, spelling backwards) are administered verbally. Particularly in individuals with a hearing impairment, this may cause test bias. For example, Thomas et al. (1983) used both a verbal measure on mental status and a non-verbal one in a sample of older individuals. While a significant relationship between hearing acuity and cognitive functioning was found for the verbally administered test, no such relationship was demonstrated with the non-verbal measure.

(cont)

Table 7.1. Outcome measures used in the studies reviewed in this chapter

Outcome measure	Domain	Reference
Activities of Daily Living Index (ADL) or Instrumental Activities of Daily Living (IADL)	Physical health	Cacciatore et al. (1999) Carabellese et al. (1993) Keller et al. (1999) Lee, Smith and Kington (1999) Luppsakko et al. (2002) Strawbridge et al. (2000)
Anxiety about Ageing Scale	Anxiety	Gomez and Madey (2001)
Attitude Toward Loss of Hearing Questionnaire (ATLHQ)	Coping	Gomez and Madey (2001)
Auditory Verbal Learning Test	Cognition	Van Boxtel et al. (2000)
Beck Anxiety Inventory	Anxiety	Andersson and Green (1995)
Beck Depression Inventory (BDI)	Depression	Carabellese et al. (1993) Knutson and Lansing (1990)
Center for Epidemiologic Studies – Depression scale (CES-D)	Depression	Kramer et al. (2002) Tesch-Römer and Nowak (1998)
Communication Profile for the Hearing Impaired (CPHI)	Communication and coping with hearing loss	Erdman and Demorest (1998a, 1998b) Gomez and Madey (2001) Garstecki and Erler (1999) Knutson and Lansing (1990)
Comprehensive Assessment and Referral Evaluation (CARE) schedule	Dementia Depression Social isolation	Gilhome Herbst and Humphrey (1980) Weinstein and Ventry (1982) Gilhome Herbst (1983)
De Jong–Gierveld Scale	Loneliness	Kramer et al. (2002)

Table 7.1. (cont)

Outcome measure	Domain	Reference
DSM-III-R	Depression	Strawbridge et al. (2000)
EuroQol	Quality of Life	Joore et al. (2003)
Eysenck Personality Inventory	Personality	Stephens (1980)
General Self-efficacy Scale	Self-efficacy	Kramer et al. (2002)
Geriatric Depression Scale	Depression	Cacciatore et al. (1999)
		Mulrow et al. (1990)
		Werngren-Elgström, Dehlin and Iwarsson (2003)
Gothenburg Profile	Hearing disability and handicap	Parving et al. (2001)
Gothenburg Quality of Life measure	Quality of Life	Werngren-Elgström, Dehlin and Iwarsson (2003)
Halstead Category test	Cognition	Thomas et al. (1983)
Health Risk Appraisal for Older Persons	Risk factors for functional impairment	Stuck et al. (2002)
Hearing Handicap Inventory for the Elderly/ Adults (HHIE)	Hearing handicap	Mulrow et al. (1990)
		Newman et al. (1997)
		Tesch-Römer and Nwak (1998)
		Wiley et al. (2000)
Hearing Measurement Scale (HMS)	Hearing disability and handicap	Karlsson-Epsmark et al. (2002)
		Thomas et al. (1983)
Intellectual function	Cognition	Lindenberger and Baltes (1994)
Interview (semi-structured, depth, audiotaped)		Aguayo and Coady (2001)
		Herth (1998)
		Karlsson-Epsmark and Hansson-Scherman (2003)
		Luey, Glass and Elliott (1995)
		Pichora-Fuller, Johnson and Roodenburg (1998)
		Rutman and Boisseau (1995)
		Salomon, Vesterager and Jagd (1988)

Instrument	Measure	Reference
Interview Schedule for Social Interaction (ISSI)		Vesterager and Salomon (1991) Vesterager, Salomon and Jagd (1988)
Jacob's Cognitive Screening Exam	Cognition	Thomas et al. (1983)
Kellner–Sheffield Symptom Questionnaire	Emotional state	Thomas et al. (1983)
Life Effects Questionnaire (open-ended)	Participation	Thomas et al. (1983)
Linn's SELF	Social relationships	Stephens, Gianopoulos and Kerr (2001) Bess (2000) Carabellese et al. (1993) Mulrow et al. (1990)
Livingston's Sleep Disturbance scale	Insomnia	Werngren-Elgström, Dehlin and Iwarsson (2003)
Louisville Older Persons Events Schedule	Stressful life events	Jang et al. (2002)
Mental Status Questionnaire (MSQ)	Cognition	Carabellese et al. (1993)
Middlesex Hospital Questionnaire	Personality	Stephens (1980)
Mini-Mental State Examination	Cognition	Bazargan, Baker and Bazargan (2001) Cacciatore et al. (1999) Naramura et al. (1999)
Minnesota Multiphasic Personality Inventory (MMPI)	Personality	Knutson and Lansing (1990)
Multidimensional Functional Assessment Questionnaire (MFAQ)	Social, economic resources Health and ADL	Marcus-Bernstein (1986)
Neo Five Factor Inventory	Neuroticism	Jang et al. (2002)
Nottingham Health Profile	Health (mental, physical)	Bess (2000) Ringdahl and Grimby (2000)
Pearlin Mastery Scale	Mastery	Kramer et al. (2002)
PHAB (Profile of Hearing Aid Benefit)	Hearing aid benefit	Scherer and Frisina (1998)
Philadelphia Geriatric Center Morale Scale (PGC)	Wellbeing	Bazargan, Baker and Bazargan (2001)

(cont)

Table 7.1. (cont)

Outcome measure	Domain	Reference
Problems Questionnaire	Problems	Stephens and Hétu (1991) Stephens, France and Lormore (1995)
Quantified Denver Scale of Communication Function	Communication	Beynon, Thornton and Poole (1997), Mulrow et al. (1990)
Rathus Assertiveness scale	Willingness to assert and engage	Knutson and Lansing (1990)
SDS (self-rating depression scale)	Depression	Naramura et al. (1999)
Self-Evaluation of Life Function (SELF)	Generic functional health	Mulrow et al. (1990)
SF-36	Health-related QoL	Parving et al. (2001)
Short Portable Mental Status Questionnaire	Cognition	Mulrow et al. (1990)
Sickness Impact Profile	Quality of life	Bess et al. (1989, 2000)
Social Anxiety and Distress (SAD) scale	Anxiety and distress	Knutson and Lansing (1990)
Social network size	Number of friends or relatives	Kramer et al. (2002) Jang et al. (2002)
Social Readjustment Rating Scale	Stressful life events	Bazargan, Baker and Bazargan (2001)
Spelling backwards	Cognition	Bazargan, Baker and Bazargan (2001)
Symptoms Check List (SCL-90)	Psychological and somatic distress.	Eriksson-Mangold and Carlsson (1991)
Ten-Flex scale	Coping	Tesch-Romer and Nowak (1998)
UCLA Loneliness Scale	Loneliness	Tesch-Römer and Nowak (1998)
Wechsler Memory Scale	Short and long term memory	Thomas et al. (1983)

Communication (d3)

Difficulty in communication is a fundamental and highly relevant limitation experienced by people with hearing loss. Communication is a broad concept. It includes understanding verbal messages, following conversations, and detecting, identifying, discriminating and localizing verbal and non-verbal sounds. Within the framework of the ICF, the disability itself (e.g. difficulty understanding speech, localizing sounds, discriminating sounds) is considered as a *limitation in activity*. A substantial amount of literature on disabilities (activity limitations) resulting from hearing impairment has been published, and recent overviews are available in Noble (1998), Bentler and Kramer (2000) and Dillon (2001).

The role of hearing and communication for a human being is essential. Ramsdell (1947) distinguished three levels of hearing:

1. The *primitive* level involves an unconscious awareness of background sounds. It gives individuals a sense of self and of being part of the environment. It has an existential value, for elderly people too (Karlsson-Epsmark and Hansson-Scherman, 2003). Loss of this primitive level may result in depression (Kampfe and Smith, 1998).
2. The second level is that of *signs or warning signals* requiring conscious awareness serving to alert the individual. Misunderstanding environmental sounds generally leads to embarrassment, fear and anxiety, and takes away the ability to enjoy sounds such as music (Smith and Kampfe, 1997).
3. The third level is the *symbolic level* which refers to communication with others. It is the level that most people relate with hearing loss. Luey, Glass and Elliott (1995) describe it as follows: 'Hearing loss affects people's lives in profound and all-encompassing ways and the most damaging thing about it is that it interferes with communication.' Noble (1996) describes linguistic communication as a capacity that enables all the various practical activities of everyday human life to be organized, sustained and accounted for. Lubinski and Welland (1997) investigated the role of communication in normal ageing elders and observed that communication is an essential tool for living safely and independently, for maintaining interests and a sense of purpose, for continuing important social and family relationships, and for exercising active control over quality of life and care.

As stated, the inability to perceive sounds and communicate within the range considered normal for a human being may affect participation in many areas of life. Each of these areas will be discussed in the following sections of this chapter.

Mobility (d4), self-care (d5), domestic life (d6)

Although it may seem unlikely that hearing impairment directly affects changing and maintaining body position, arm use, washing, dressing or moving and lifting objects, the effect of auditory impairment on self-care and domestic life has been demonstrated in a number of studies (Carabellese et al., 1993; Cacciatore et al., 1999; Lee, Smith and Kington, 1999; Strawbridge et al., 2000). The outcome measure used in these studies was the Activities of Daily Living (ADL) index, a standardized measure of daily life activities. Participants were asked if they had difficulty in bathing, dressing, eating, getting in and out of bed or rising from a chair, and using the toilet. At an increased level of hearing loss, a lower ADL score (reflecting a reduction of functional status) was recorded, independent of visual acuity and after controlling for age, gender and socio-economic status. Despite the fact that cognition was the most important factor in one of these studies predicting ADL, a significant independent effect of hearing was shown (Carabellese et al., 1993). Using the Sickness Impact Profile (SIP), Bess and co-workers (1989) demonstrated an association between hearing loss and the physical scale (combining ambulation, mobility, body care and movement).

In a longitudinal study, Wallhagen (1996) found that hearing-impaired elderly people – at a 6-year follow-up – were significantly more likely to just sit down and do nothing than those with no hearing impairment.

Bumin et al. (2002) found hearing problems to be one of the risk factors for falling among frail elderly people in a Turkish rest home (Bumin et al., 2002). There is quite an extensive literature on balance problems and falls in elderly people. Balance problems frequently occur as a result of the same pathology that causes the hearing problems.

It must be mentioned here that the ADL is in fact located in the domain of *activity limitation* rather than in the domain of *participation restriction*. There is, however, no doubt about the high likelihood that limitations in daily life activities such as mobility, self-care and domestic life may have a major impact on participation in life.

Although the above studies assert a relationship between deteriorated hearing and restrictions in mobility, self-care and domestic life, conflicting evidence is found in other studies. For example, Mulrow and colleagues (1990) examined group differences (hearing vs hearing-impaired) and did not observe an effect of hearing loss on the Self-Evaluation of Life Function (SELF), a generic measure of quality of life, including physical disability. The lack of sensitivity and appropriateness of various generic measures of quality of life, usually including physical disability scales, to be used for assessing the impact of hearing loss are discussed further by Bess (2000) and Parving et al. (2001).

Interpersonal interactions and relations (d7)

There is no doubt that hearing loss affects interpersonal interactions and relations as a result of alterations in the ability to communicate. Hearing impairment hinders communication with others, either directly or indirectly. Smith and Kampfe (1997) give an overview of basic interpersonal/relationship implications of hearing loss for older people. These include changes in family dynamics as a result of misconceptions, misunderstanding, the need to repeat, changes in family roles and independent functioning (spouses become caregivers). Further implications are fatigue or decrease in energy as a result of compensatory strategies, isolation, decreased recreational outlets, anxiety, fear, distrust and the presumption by others that the older person is experiencing cognitive deterioration. These findings have also been reported in whole or in part by others (Stephens, France and Lormore, 1995; Herth, 1998; Aguayo and Coady, 2001). Using the Hearing Handicap Inventory for the Elderly (HHIE), Mulrow et al. (1990) and Newman et al. (1997) emphasized the adverse relationship between hearing loss and emotional effects, such as feeling *stupid*, *dumb* or *upset*. In a review article on autobiographical reports of late-deafened adults, Rutman and Boisseau (1995) state that the reduced social contacts outside the home may result in increased time spent at home and an increased level of stress.

Also, Smith and Kampfe (1997) report an association between impaired hearing and depression. While depression may be considered as a personal/psychological factor within the ICF framework, the effect on interpersonal relationships may be strongly mediated by depression resulting from hearing loss, particularly in older age. Interpersonal functioning is traditionally altered in the presence of depression (Smith and Kampfe, 1997). Therefore, studies describing the connection between hearing loss and depression are reviewed in this section rather than under 'Psychological factors' elsewhere in this chapter.

The relationship between decreased hearing and depression has long been observed both in qualitative and in controlled studies using a variety of outcome measures (Gilhome Herbst and Humphrey, 1980; Gilhome Herbst, 1983; Vesterager, Salomon and Jagd, 1988; Vesterager and Salomon, 1991; Carabellese et al., 1993; Wallhagen, 1996; Cacciatore et al., 1999; Stephens, Gianopoulos and Kerr, 2001; Heine and Browning, 2002; Kramer et al., 2002; Werngren-Elgström, Dehlin and Iwarsson, 2003). In a systematic investigation of older adults (50–102 years), Strawbridge et al. (2000) explored the longitudinal impact of two levels of self-reported hearing impairment on a number of health variables, adjusting for co-morbid conditions and other confounding variables, such as age, gender and education. Depression, self-rated mental health and social functioning changed negatively in a dose-response pattern for those with progressive levels of hearing impairment compared with those reporting no impairment.

Another psychosocial factor related to restricted participation in interpersonal interactions and relations due to hearing loss is loneliness. In a study by Knutson and Lansing (1990), pervasive loneliness was observed among severely impaired candidates for cochlear implantation. The results not only showed high and significant correlations between communication difficulties at home (Communication Profile for the Hearing Impaired or CPHI) and scores on the UCLA loneliness scale, but also that the hard-of-hearing participants were comparable to the loneliest groups of people with whom the UCLA loneliness scale was ever used. Apparently, limitations in the activity to communicate, particularly in intimate settings, have great impact on feelings of loneliness among those with profound hearing loss.

Further corroboration of the relationship between hearing loss and loneliness has been established in both qualitative and controlled studies (Gilhome Herbst, 1983; Herth, 1998; Strawbridge et al., 2000; Kramer et al., 2002).

One further reflection of participation restriction in interpersonal interactions is the number of friends relative to the past (Gilhome Herbst, 1983) or the size of the present social network, a determinant of psychosocial functioning in elderly people used in a study by Kramer et al. (2002). Gilhome Herbst (1983) found hearing-impaired elderly people more likely to say they have fewer friends than in the past, compared to normally hearing elderly people. The sample in Kramer's study included 3107 older adults with ages ranging from 55 to 85 years. Social network size was defined as the number of adults with whom somebody maintains an important and regular relationship (household members, children, parents, other family member, neighbours, colleagues, others). Hearing loss appeared to be significantly associated with the size of the social network, those with hearing loss having a smaller social network than their hearing peers. A remarkable finding was the absence of association between presence of a number of chronic diseases (cancer, cardiac disease, diabetes, stroke, lung disease, arthritis) and size of the social network. This result emphasizes the importance of hearing loss in psychosocial health assessment in elderly people.

Although several investigators demonstrate an overall negative effect of hearing impairment on psychosocial health, some studies failed to demonstrate this relationship. An example is the study of Mulrow et al. (1990), who found no significant effect of deteriorated hearing on depression in their cross-sectional study. Although depression appeared to be more prevalent in the group of elderly people with hearing loss (compared to those without hearing impairment), the significant association between hearing loss and depression disappeared when the authors adjusted for potential confounders such as age and visual acuity.

Vesterager and Salomon (1991) studied the psychosocial impact of hearing loss among elderly people (70–75 years). They observed no significant effect of hearing loss on loneliness when comparing hearing-impaired elderly people with normally hearing peers. Thomas et al. (1983) failed to demonstrate an association between hearing loss and depression and measures of social interaction. Finally, Eriksson-Mangold and Carlsson (1991) did not find a significant correlation between experienced disability and handicap (HMS) and depression.

Major life events (d8)

According to the ICF framework, major life events include education, work, employment and economic transactions. These issues have scarcely been investigated in studies focusing on elderly people. Kampfe and Smith (1998) report a lack of ability among older adults with hearing loss to make truly informed financial decisions. Most samples in studies on elderly people comprise groups of retired people. Whenever questions on work are included in studies among samples with a wide range of ages, work is considered as not applicable for the older part of the sample. A detailed review of the importance of work for psychosocial health is described in the previous chapter of this book.

Community, social and civic life (d9)

Participation in community, social and civic life comprises actions and tasks required to engage in organized social life outside the family. Areas in which restrictions in participation may be experienced are community life, recreation and leisure, religion and spirituality, human rights, political life and citizenship (ICF: WHO, 2001).

Although hearing loss in older age may have great impact on domestic life and relationships within the family (see previous section), participation restrictions experienced in a broader social context may even be more distinct. Various studies give rise to this assumption. Using the open-ended Life Effects Questionnaire (LEQ), Stephens, Gianopoulos and Kerr (2001) observed that, when asked to list restrictions in participation, most subjects referred to the influence of the people around the person with the hearing loss in broad terms of acquaintances, neighbours, peers, etc., rather than specifying their immediate family members. Stephens (1996) concluded that the extent of the psychosocial problems an individual may experience depends on whether they act within the family or in a broader context such as in social or civic life outside the family. A respondent in a study by Karlsson-Epsmark and Hansson-Scherman (2003) reported similar findings: 'the effect of difficulties with conversation depends entirely on where you are and who you are talking to'. Comparable results were found by Aguayo and Coady (2001) in a qualitative study on the experiences of deafened adults. General oppression, exclusion and social isolation in the community are a common experience of adults with late-onset hearing loss. 'Acquired profound hearing loss causes embarrassment and fear. It makes the persons feel inadequate and incompetent to engage in social situations and civic life.' The eight respondents in Aguayo's study reported using strategies of social withdrawal or selective avoidance of anxiety-provoking situations, leading to further isolation. Additionally, Tesch-Römer and Nowak (1998) reported that coping strategies used by a person with hearing difficulties differ when the interaction occurs within the family or outside the family (see also Brooks, Hallam and Mellor, 2001). An illustration of the above findings is given in a review paper by Rutman and Boisseau (1995): 'Noisy places become hostile zones and social withdrawal seems to be the ultimate choice of deafened older adults.'

When looking at community, social and civic life, a number of studies focused on specific domains as categorized by the ICF. Ringdahl and Grimby (2000) used the Nottingham Health Profile to investigate the health-related quality of life of 311 Swedish adults with severe–profound hearing loss. A relationship between the degree of hearing loss and partici-pating in hobbies and interests and going on holiday was demonstrated, those with severe loss being less active in exploring free time compared to hearing controls. Strawbridge et al. (2000) found that those with moderate–severe hearing loss reported having 'little enjoyment of free time'. Likewise, Wallhagen (1996) reported that older adults with a hearing impairment were significantly more likely not to enjoy their free time a lot compared to those without a hearing loss. Gilhome Herbst (1983) found hearing-impaired elderly people less likely to be able to get out without help compared to normally hearing older adults.

In the longitudinal study by Strawbridge, social functioning included three variables: 'not feeling close to others', 'feeling left out even in a group' and 'feeling lonely or remote'. Social functioning decreased for those with progressive levels of hearing impairment compared with those reporting no impairment.

The HHIE covers some areas of social and civic life (e.g. shopping, attending religious services, meeting new people). Using this outcome instrument, Newman et al. (1997) found negative effects of hearing loss on wider social life, regardless of the severity of the loss. Mulrow et al. (1990) reported a relation-ship between the severity of the hearing loss and scores on the HHIE.

Finally, Karlsson-Epsmark et al. (2002) used a shortened version of the Hearing Measurement Scale, including 4 items (out of 20) on so-called quality of life (I enjoy sounds in nature/music; I avoid meeting people; I avoid going to theatre). In a sample of 154 older adults with acquired hearing loss (median age 77 years) no negative effect of hearing impairment on 'quality of life' was found.

With regard to community life, it is important to consider the difference between the culturally (or prelingually) Deaf and hard-of-hearing (or deafened) people. Luey, Glass and Elliott (1995) describe the discrepancy between the two groups. The Deaf tend to perceive deafness not as a disability, but rather as an alternative lifestyle and culture with its own sign language, whereas for the deafened it is both a disability and a loss. People who have been affiliated primarily with the speaking and hearing world are generally seen as strangers or aliens in the Deaf community (Luey, Glass and Elliott, 1995). As a consequence, the two groups may differ in political aspirations. While hard-of-hearing people may put effort into making assistive listening devices available in public areas, the Deaf organizations may be active in promoting acceptance of sign language and the rights and abilities of the Deaf. The agenda of the hard-of-hearing groups may be unrelated to sign language, which may be seen by the Deaf community as a threat to their language and culture (Luey, Glass and Elliott, 1995).

Society's attitude towards deafness and deafened people must be viewed as a critical ecological variable affecting self-identity, self-esteem and adjustment processes (Rutman and Boisseau, 1995). The authors emphasize the importance of considering these matters in rehabilitation settings.

Environmental factors

Support and relationships (e3)

The significant other

In the ecological approach to hearing disability (activity limitation) and handicap (participation restriction), the role of the significant other, in influencing the developing psychosocial difficulties an individual with hearing loss may experience, has been clearly demonstrated (Noble and Hétu, 1994; Stephens, 1996; Borg, 1998). Elsewhere in this book, Stephens describes the two-way interaction between the individual with the hearing loss and the significant other: while the attitude and approach of those around them will affect the impact of hearing loss on the patient, the patient's problems will impact on those around them.

Hearing loss is invisible and is therefore frequently misunderstood. Inappropriate tactics of hearing people and negative attitudes towards people with hearing impairments may have a more negative impact on the patient than the hearing loss itself (Strong and Shaver, 1991; Rutman and Boisseau, 1995). Noble (1996) emphasizes the features that promote the undesirability of the status of being hearing-impaired. Overgeneralization, stereotyping and prejudices by others motivate the person with the hearing loss to avoid being identified by others – or to self-identify – as having impaired hearing. Particularly among elderly people, a common experience is the feeling of being left out of conversations and discussion as a result of the assumption that the cognitive capacities are reduced, while in fact only hearing acuity is affected. It is the sense of being undervalued that is experienced when discussion and conversations are simplified and/or reduced (also due to effort and fatigue) and does not reflect the intellectual capacities of the older person with hearing impairment (Rutman and Boisseau, 1995; Smith and Kampfe, 1997).

Stephens (1996) highlights the link between the compensatory role of the significant other and the psychosocial health of the person with the hearing loss. The death or departure of a spouse may make the individual aware of hearing difficulties and participation restrictions when the partner is no longer available, for example to answer the phone or doorbell or to steer the impaired individual through conversations.

For many older adults and particularly for the oldest-old, the role of the significant other may be fulfilled by a nurse, a doctor or another staff member in a nursing home or other hospital setting. Hines (2000) and Fooks et al. (2000) addressed the inadequate training of both nurses and doctors in deaf awareness and associated communication skills, causing difficulties and disadvantages for patients with hearing impairment.

Support

The role of support is an important one. In a study on determinants of self-perceived hearing problems among older adults, Jang et al. (2002) found that emotional support results in a more positive perception of hearing problems.

Personal factors

The classification used in Chapter 5 is followed here, and the key areas are highlighted in Table 7.2.

Gender

Except for the documentation of gender differences in the age-related loss of sensitivity to a pure tone (Jerger et al., 1993; Pearson et al., 1995; Parving et al., 1997), relatively little is known about gender differences in the impact of hearing loss on psychosocial health in older age. So far, there have been a

Table 7.2. A classification of personal contextual factors, based on the ICF (2001). Areas of interest in the present context are indicated in bold type

Gender, race, age	**Education**
Other health conditions	Profession
Fitness	**Past and current experience**
Lifestyle	Overall behaviour pattern and character style
Habits	**– Fatigue, energy**
– Addictions	Individual psychological assets
Upbringing	**– Personality/emotions**
Coping styles	
Social background	

relatively small number of contributions to this area of research (Kricos, 2000). Using the CPHI, Garstecki and Erler (1999) investigated self-perceived hearing handicap among men and women with acquired mild–moderate sensorineural hearing loss, aged 65 years and older, living independently. Controlling for demographic variables (income, education, intelligence, ego strength, general health, employment status, marital status) and hearing (better ear four-frequency average pure-tone audiogram [PTA]), significant gender differences were noted for six scales. Compared to men with a hearing impairment, women with hearing loss assigned greater importance to effective social communication, were more likely to use non-verbal communication strategies, and reported greater anxiety and stress, greater problem awareness and less denial associated with hearing loss. These results confirmed the findings of Erdman and Demorest (1998a, 1998b) who included participants with a wider range of ages (16–97 years, median age 68.4 years, mean age 64.4 years). Weak correlations between gender and certain CPHI scales were observed: women placed greater importance than men on communication in social situations, reported more frequent use of non-verbal strategies and were lower in areas of personal adjustment.

In a community survey with 5145 participants, Stephens, Lewis and Charny (1991) applied the Problem Questionnaire. Among the 625 respondents reporting any auditory problems a significant age/gender interaction effect was found in the 60–70 year olds, men showing greater problems than women. Using the Nottingham Health Profile, Ringdahl and Grimby (2000) observed lower quality-of-life scores of women with hearing impairment, compared to men. Vesterager and Salomon (1991) observed a higher incidence of adverse coping reactions (e.g. pretending to hear and withdrawal) among men compared to women with hearing loss.

Race, ethnicity

Most studies on psychosocial functioning among elderly people have been conducted in predominantly white populations. The issue of race or ethnicity and its relationship with the impact of hearing loss on psychosocial health status have been addressed in a few studies, which are – to my knowledge – all focused on African–American minority groups. Bazargan, Baker and Bazargan (2001) conducted a study on the association between sensory impairments and subjective wellbeing among aged African–Americans. Compared to the general population, higher prevalence rates of visual and hearing impairment were observed. An indirect negative effect of hearing loss (mediated by functional status) on wellbeing was found. A remarkable outcome was the underutilization of audiological care: only 4.3% of those reporting poor hearing wore hearing aids.

Marcus-Bernstein (1986) explored the role of audiological and non-audiological measures in relation to handicap in a sample of 100 black elderly people (aged >65 years) with mild–severe sensorineural hearing loss. Besides audiological measures, dependability (a dimension of the social support scale MFAQ) and lethargy and paranoid (mental health subscale) emerged as contributing predictors for psychosocial health, measured by means of the HHIE and the Hearing Measurement Scale.

Erdman and Demorest (1998a, 1998b) considered race or ethnicity as a potential confounder in a study of 1008 subjects (76% > 55 years) on adjustment to hearing loss and distinguished six categories: white (82.6%), black (10.4%), Hispanic (2.6%), Asian (3.2%), Alaskan (0.5%) and multiple ethnicities (0.7%). The CPHI was used as an outcome measure. Race/ethnicity was significantly related to only two scales: communication performance in average situations and problem awareness. Better performance and greater problem awareness was observed among whites than among African–Americans.

Regardless of race/ethnicity, cultural differences may further influence the impact of hearing loss on the psychosocial difficulties that an individual may experience. In this respect it is interesting to examine the results of comparable studies performed in different parts of the world. A search of the literature yielded a list of roughly equivalent (population) studies conducted in the countries shown in Table 7.3. A remarkable outcome is that essentially similar results were obtained. In each of those studies, hearing loss had a significant adverse effect on one or more different determinants of psychosocial functioning or was an important indicator of psychosocial health among elderly people. While type and degree of psychosocial distress may differ, hearing loss seems to be a universally relevant indicator of psychosocial health.

Table 7.3. Psychosocial studies from different countries

China	Chou and Chi (2002)
Denmark	Vesterager and Salomon (1991)
Finland	Lupsakko, Mäntyjärvi and Kautiainen (2002)
Germany	Stuck et al. (2002); Tesch-Römer (1997)
Italy	Cacciatore et al. (1999); Carabellese et al. (1993)
Japan	Naramura et al. (1999)
Netherlands	Kramer et al. (2002),
Sweden	Ringdahl and Grimby (2000); Sixt and Rosenhall (1997)
Switzerland	Stuck et al. (2002)
Turkey	Bumin et al. (2002)
UK	Stephens, Gianopoulos and Kerr (2001); Stuck et al. (2002)
USA	Bazargan, Baker and Bazargan (2001); Lee, Smith and Kington (1999); Mulrow et al. (1990); Strawbridge et al. (2000); Wallhagen (1996)

Other health conditions

In older age, co-morbidity is a crucial issue in research on the psychosocial health status and quality of life. It is a notorious confounder. Although hearing loss is frequently perceived as a normal life event, for older adults decreased acuity in hearing comes at a time when multiple losses may be occurring simultaneously and when social, psychological and financial resources may also be declining (Rutman and Boisseau, 1995).

As described in the previous sections, several investigators have documented and controlled for co-morbidity, showing an independent adverse effect of hearing on psychosocial health (Mulrow et al., 1990; Strawbridge et al., 2000). Co-morbid medical status was also controlled for in a study by Kramer et al. (2002). Determinants of psychosocial functioning in this study were depression, mastery (controlling one's own life vs fatalistically ruled), self-efficacy, loneliness and social network size. An independent adverse effect of hearing loss was found. Moreover, except for depression, hearing loss appeared to have a greater negative association with psychosocial health than did other chronic conditions such as cancer, diabetes, cardiac disease and peripheral arterial disease.

The existence of age-related vision and hearing loss and the likely interactive effect on participation in life are addressed in a number of studies. Lee, Smith and Kington (1999) and Carabellese et al. (1993) found vision and hearing independently related to decrements in functional status (ADL) and wellbeing. A dose–response pattern was observed. The extent of decreased functioning rose in response to the deterioration in the self-rated quality of the sense of function. Lupsakko, Mäntyjärvi and Kautiainen (2002) investigated the effect of combined visual and hearing impairment on activities in daily living, and found a decrease in ADL functions only in those with combined impairment. Keller et al. (1999) reported similar findings: combined vision and hearing impairments have greater effect on functional status (ADL) than single sensory impairments and the influence is independent of mental status and co-morbid illnesses.

Coping

Is it the hearing impairment *per se*, or is it the inadequate coping behaviour causing poor psychosocial functioning? There is growing evidence for the latter. Various investigators addressed the issue of coping in older adults with hearing loss, the vast majority using the CPHI. Gomez and Madey (2001) administered both the verbal and non-verbal adaptive strategies subscales (e.g. hearing aids, facing the person, asking others to talk louder, repeat, talk slower and face you, situating yourself to hear the speaker better and amplification devices) and the maladaptive behaviours subscale (pretending to understand, interrupting conversations, avoiding talking to strangers, avoiding social situations, dominating conversations and ignoring the speaker). The sample comprised 61 adults, aged 61–85 years (mean 75.5). Two simultaneous regression analyses were conducted, one predicting the use of adaptive strategies and one predicting the use of maladaptive strategies. The use of adaptive strategies was predicted by perceived effectiveness of strategies. The use of maladaptive strategies was predicted by perceived effectiveness of strategies, poor adjustment to hearing loss and poor social support (the last two variables measured by the Attitude Toward Loss of Hearing Questionnaire – ALTHQ). Although physical hearing loss (PTA) was included in both analyses, it did not contribute significantly in the prediction of coping strategies.

In a small sample of 27 profoundly impaired participants (aged 22–71 years), Knutson and Lansing (1990) calculated correlations between communication difficulties (CPHI scores) and seven general measures of psychological functioning: loneliness, depression, social isolation, anxiety, lack of assertiveness and suspicion. Communication strategies and adjustment to hearing loss (CPHI) – rather than the communication difficulties *per se* – appeared to correlate to depression, loneliness, anxiety in social settings and lack of assertiveness. It must be noted here that, although the authors gave a detailed overview of 'age of onset of hearing loss' and 'years of hearing aid use', adjustments for these potential co-variables were not made.

Tesch-Römer and Nowak (1998) observed similar findings in a study among 79 older adults with hearing loss (aged 54–86 years, mean 71 years). The TEN-Flex scale was applied to measure evasive (passive and avoiding) and invasive (active and intervening) coping strategies. Correlation patterns showed no relationship between coping strategies and the degree of hearing loss (better ear average [BEA] 0.5, 1, 2 kHz), while evasive coping strategies were significantly related to depression and loneliness.

Social background and education

The impact of socio-economic status on the adverse impact of loss of senses on hearing has frequently been demonstrated and is therefore controlled for in most studies investigating the association between hearing and psychosocial health. Sixt and Rosenhall (1997) highlighted the role of socio-economic factors affecting health among older adults in terms of access to health care. Some critical researchers postulate the role of socio-economic status as the one and only relevant factor in hearing (Hinchcliffe, 1990). However, in a large controlled study of 7320 elderly people (aged > 70 years) by Lee, Smith and Kington (1999), adjustment for socio-economic status added little compared with the adjustment for health conditions and demographic variables. The authors argue that their findings are an illustration of the universality of the adverse effect of hearing loss on patients' wellbeing across socio-economic groups. Their conclusion is that psychosocial difficulties exist, regardless of economic status.

As is the case for socio-economic status, education is frequently found to be an important confounding variable in studies on the interrelationship of hearing, psychosocial functioning and adjustment to hearing loss. Various investigators have shown a significant relationship, those with higher levels of education reporting better hearing, better communication performance and less frequent use of maladaptive behavioural strategies (Gatehouse, 1990; Sixt and Rosenhall, 1997; Erdman and Demorest, 1998a, 1998b).

Past and current experience

Jang et al. (2002) investigated the role of stressful life events on self-perceived hearing among 425 older adults (aged 60–85 years). Examples of such events are new illnesses or injuries, death of significant others and reduction in income. Participants in Jang's study were asked to report if certain events had occurred within the past 12 months. Controlling for demographic variables and screened hearing, stressful life events explained an additional 3% of the variance in the hierarchical regression model for self-perceived hearing problems.

Stephens, Lewis and Charny (1991) and Rosenhall et al. (1993) highlighted the role of smoking. Smokers seem to complain more about hearing difficulties than non-smokers.

Overall behaviour pattern and character style

Fatigue, energy

Fatigue, energy and mental effort may result from behavioural modifications by the individual with the hearing loss which may reduce the primary restriction in participation, but, in turn, may result in a secondary handicap because of the effort involved in such a process. This phenomenon has been highlighted in several studies (Hétu et al., 1988; Kramer et al., 1997; Smith and Kampfe, 1997; Herth, 1998; Kampfe and Smith, 1998; Ringdahl and Grimby, 2000). Werngren-Elgström, Dehlin and Iwarsson (2003) compared a group of prelingual deaf elderly people with a similar age group of adults needing rehabilitation other than hearing rehabilitation. Although general fatigue (Gothenburg Quality of Life) was equally present in both groups, insomnia (Livingston's sleep disturbance scale) appeared to be more frequent among prelingually deaf elderly people.

Individual psychological assets

Personality/emotions

Like the two-way interaction of the impaired individual with the significant other, a mutual relationship exists between the individual with the hearing loss and their personality: the personality of the person may influence the response to hearing loss, while the (acquired) hearing loss and its consequences may affect the personality of the patient. Intrapersonal changes (those within the self) that may occur among older adults with acquired hearing loss are highlighted by Kampfe and Smith (1998). Among the losses associated with late-onset hearing impairment are the loss of sense of self, loss of sense of safety, loss of enjoyment of environmental sounds and music, and loss of easy interaction with others. Kampfe and Smith (1998) distinguish various emotional states (responses) associated with hearing loss. Among them are shock, realization, defensive retreat, acknowledgement and adaptation. Depression is also considered as an emotional state. (The relationship between hearing deterioration and depression has been addressed elsewhere in this chapter.)

The issue of hearing loss affecting self-identity and self-esteem has been raised by various investigators (Rutman and Boisseau, 1995; Herth, 1998; Karlsson-Epsmark and Hansson-Scherman, 2003). Mulrow et al. (1990) observed a borderline significant adverse effect ($p < 0.07$) of hearing loss on the self-esteem SELF subscale. Rutman and Boisseau (1995) describe the changes in perceived autonomy and the tandem principle with regard to self-identity: changes in self-identity of the hearing-impaired individual may change the self-identity of the significant other as well (e.g. from wife to caregiver).

It must be noted here that Vesterager, Salomon and Jagd (1988) did not observe a significant effect of hearing loss on self-assessed mood and self-esteem when comparing hearing-impaired elderly people with normally hearing peers.

Jang et al. (2002) explored the role of neuroticism as a determinant of self-perceived hearing difficulties among older adults (60–84 years). Individuals with a higher level of neuroticism had a more adverse perception of their hearing problems. Using the Eysenck Personality Inventory and the Middlesex Hospital Questionnaire, Stephens (1980) found elevated levels of neuroticism and introversion in the hearing-impaired sample compared to a normal population.

Knutson and Lansing (1990) used the Minnesota Multiphasic Personality Inventory (MMPI) to assess enduring personality patterns among profoundly impaired adults (20–71 years) and found limited communication performance at home (CPHI) to be related to social introversion. No correlation was found between communication difficulties and suspiciousness (scale 6 of the MMPI).

Eriksson-Mangold and Carlsson (1991) investigated the occurrence of psychological and somatic distress in people with acquired hearing loss in a sample of older adults (55–74 years). They observed significant relationships between speech recognition and various dimensions of the Symptoms Checklist (SCL-90): anxiety, hostility, paranoid ideation and psychoticism. The association between anxiety and hearing loss in elderly people was also addressed by Andersson and Green (1995). These authors argue that the adverse effect of hearing loss on anxiety may be mediated by depression.

Other factors

Profound–severe vs mild–moderate hearing loss; congenital vs acquired

Evidence exists about the discrepancy between pure-tone hearing loss and the type and extent of limitations and restrictions an individual may experience in daily life. Even if the degree of hearing loss according to the PTA is minimal, the effects on psychosocial functioning and quality of life may be manifest, and vice versa. Many studies have been published on this topic (Eriksson-Mangold and Carlsson, 1991; Kramer et al., 1996; Newman et al., 1997; Scherer and Frisina, 1998; Pichora-Fuller, Johnson and Roodenburg, 1998; Karlsson-Epsmark et al., 2002). Self-reported hearing seems to be a more adequate assessment of difficulties experienced in daily life. In general, linear relationships are observed between the degree of self-assessed hearing difficulty and the severity of psychosocial problems, those with severe–profound hearing loss having greater psychosocial dysfunction than those with milder losses (Knutson and Lansing, 1990; Carabellese et al., 1993; Lee et al., 1999; Strawbridge et al., 2000).

In most studies reviewed in this chapter, the aetiology of the hearing loss has not been considered and information about time of onset of hearing loss is rarely available. The great majority of the investigations covered in this review include participants who have an acquired hearing loss. It may be assumed that among elderly people the type of hearing loss is predominantly sensorineural. Kampfe and Smith (1998) report relevant considerations within this respect: sensorineural losses – as opposed to conductive losses – do not just result in a reduction of loudness, but signals are experienced in a distorted way. This may result in differential hearing (i.e. seeming to hear sometimes and not at other times), which is frequently misunderstood by family members and others. It must be noted here that Gatehouse and Haggard (1987) have published evidence suggesting that at low stimulus levels people with conductive hearing loss suffer greater disability (in terms of word recognition) than people with sensorineural hearing loss.

Literature on the psychosocial effects among Deaf elderly people is scarce. Most studies on Deafness deal with children and adolescents. An exception is the study by Werngren-Elgström, Dehlin and Iwarsson (2003). They investigated subjective wellbeing and the prevalence of depressive symptoms and insomnia among prelingually Deaf older adults using sign language. Scores on the Gothenburg Quality of Life (GQL), the Geriatric Depression Scale (GDS) and the Livingston sleep disturbance scale were compared with similar age groups of hearing elderly people. Although depressive symptoms and insomnia occurred more frequently among the prelingually Deaf people, no difference between the groups for subjective wellbeing was observed.

Effect of rehabilitation on psychosocial functioning

Literature on the effect of hearing aids on psychosocial health status is relatively scarce. Available data suggest that fitting of hearing aids is a successful treatment for enhancing psychosocial wellbeing and reversing the deterioration in the quality of life. Joore and colleagues (2003) examined the effect of fitting hearing aids among 80 first-time hearing aid users (aged 28–95 years, mean 68 years) with mild–moderate hearing loss. Among the outcome measures were the EuroQoL and the SF-36. No effect on generic quality of life (EuroQoL) was determined, but hearing aid fitting did improve social functioning (SF-36). The National Council on the Aging (NCOA, 1999) studied the consequences of untreated hearing loss in older people, as well as the benefits of hearing-aid fitting, in a sample of 2304 adults aged 50 years and older. Both individuals with hearing loss and their significant others were included. Controlling for age, gender and income, the results showed that those who did not use hearing aids were more likely to report sadness, depression, worry, anxiety, paranoia, less social activity and insecurity. Family members were even more likely to report improvements in terms of relationships at home, feelings about themselves, life overall and relationships with children and grandchildren.

Among those having hearing problems in a study by Cacciatore et al. (1999), older people with hearing aids had fewer depressive symptoms than hearing-impaired participants without hearing aids. A positive association between hearing aids and cognition was also observed.

In a 6-month follow-up study by Tesch-Römer (1997), a group of elderly first-time hearing-aid users was compared with two age-matched control groups (hearing-impaired people without hearing aids and a normally hearing group). While hearing aids appeared to have a positive effect on self-perceived handicap, no effect of hearing aids on social activities, satisfaction with social relations, well-being or cognitive functioning was observed. Stephens, Vetter and Lewis (2003) highlighted the minor influence of hearing aids on the considerable difficulties elderly people experience in common activities and communication situations. Further reviews by Bess (2000) and Arlinger (2003) reported positive effects of amplification on various measures of quality of life and cognition.

Besides hearing aids, other types of rehabilitation may improve the psychosocial health status of elderly people. Examples of such interventions are hearing tactics, lip-reading, communication courses and active listening training (Kricos and Holmes, 1996; Beynon, Thornton and Poole, 1997; Kricos, 1997; Hickson and Worrall, 2003).

Fooks et al. (2000) assessed the patient's satisfaction with communication with their medical staff and studied the effect of acetate cards above the beds of in-hospital patients and voice amplifiers among 200 older hospital inpatients (70–97 years). Before the intervention, 22% of the patients rated communication with their doctor as unsatisfactory. A significant enhancement (reduction of problems to 6%) was reached after using voice amplifiers and acetate cards.

References

Aguayo MO, Coady NF (2001) The experience of deafened adults: implications for rehabilitative services. Health and Social Work 26: 269–276.

Andersson G, Green M (1995) Anxiety in elderly hearing impaired persons. Perceptual and Motor Skills 81: 552–554.

Arlinger S (2003) Negative consequences of uncorrected hearing loss – a review. International Journal of Audiology 42(suppl 2): S17–S20.

Bazargan J, Baker S, Bazargan SH (2001) Sensory impairments and subjective well-being among aged African American persons. Journal of Gerontology, Psychological Sciences 56B: 268–278.

Bentler RA, Kramer SE (2000) Guidelines for choosing a self-report outcome measure. Ear and Hearing 21: S37–49.

Bess FH (2000) The role of generic health-related quality of life measures in establishing audiological rehabilitation outcomes. Ear and Hearing 21: S74–S79.

Bess FH, Lichtenstein MJ, Logan SA, Burger MC, Nelson E (1989) Hearing impairment as a determinant of function in the elderly. Journal of the American Geriatrics Society 37: 123–128.

Beynon GJ, Thornton FL, Poole C (1997) A randomised controlled trial of the efficacy of a communication course for first time hearing aid users. British Journal of Audiology 31: 345–351.

Borg E (1998) Audiology in an ecological perspective; development of a conceptual framework. Scandinavian Audiology, Supplementum 49: 132–139.

Boxtel MPJ van, Beijsterveldt CEM van, Houx PJ et al. (2000) Mild hearing impairment can reduce verbal memory performance in a healthy adult population. Journal of Clinical and Experimental Neuropsychology 22: 147–154.

Brooks DN, Hallam RS, Mellor PA (2001) The effects on significant others of providing a hearing aid to the hearing impaired partner. British Journal of Audiology 35: 165–171.

Bumin G, Uyanik M, Aki E, Kayihan H (2002) An investigation of risk factors for frail elderly people in a Turkish rest home. Aging Clinical Experience Research 14: 192–196.

Cacciatore F, Napoli C, Abete P et al. (1999) Quality of life determinants and hearing function in an elderly population: Osservatorio Geriatrico Campano study group. Gerontology 45: 323–328.

Carabellese C, Appollonio I, Rozzini R et al. (1993) Sensory impairment (visual and hearing) and quality of life in a community elderly population. Journal of the American Geriatrics Society 41: 401–407.

Chou KL, Chi I (2002) Successful aging among the young-old, old-old and oldest-old Chinese. International Journal of Aging and Human Development 54: 1–14.

Dillon H (2001) Hearing Aids. Boomerang Press, Sydney.

Erdman SA, Demorest ME (1998a) Adjustment to hearing impairment I: description of a heterogeneous clinical population. Journal of Speech, Language and Hearing Research 41: 107–122.

Erdman SA, Demorest ME (1998b) Adjustment to hearing impairment II: audiological and demographic correlates. Journal of Speech, Language and Hearing Research 41: 123–136.

Eriksson-Mangold M, Carlsson SG (1991) Psychological and somatic distress in relation to perceived hearing disability, hearing handicap and hearing measurements. Journal of Psychosomatic Research 35: 729–740.

Fooks L, Morgan R, Sharma P, Adekoke A, Turnbull CJ (2000) The impact of hearing on communication. Postgraduate Medicine 76: 92–95.

Garstecki DC, Erler SF (1999) Older adult performance on the communication profile for the hearing impaired: gender difference. Journal of Speech, Language and Hearing Research 42: 785–796.

Gatehouse S (1990) The role of non-auditory factors in measured and self-reported disability. Acta Otolaryngologica Supplementum 476: 249–256.

Gatehouse S, Haggard MP (1987) The effects of air-bone gap and presentation level on word identification. Ear and Hearing 8: 140–146.

Gilhome Herbst K (1983) Psychosocial consequences of disorders of hearing in the elderly. In: Hinchcliffe R (ed.) Hearing and Balance. Churchill Livingstone, Edinburgh, UK, pp. 174–200.

Gilhome Herbst K, Humphrey C (1980) Hearing impairment and mental state in the elderly living at home. British Medical Journal 281: 903–905.

Gomez RW, Madey SF (2001) Coping-with-hearing-loss model for older adults. Journal of Gerontology, Psychological Sciences 56B: 223–225.

Heine C, Browning CJ (2002) Communication and psychosocial consequences of sensory loss in older adults: overview and rehabilitation directions. Disability and Rehabilitation 24: 763–773.

Herth K (1998) Integrating hearing loss into one's life. Qualitative Health Research 8: 207–223.

Hétu R, Riverin L, Lalande N, Getty L, St-Cyr C (1988) Qualitative analysis of the handicap associated with occupation hearing loss. British Journal of Audiology 22: 251–264.

Hickson L, Worrall L (2003) Beyond hearing aid fitting: Improving communication for older adults. International Journal of Audiology 42(suppl 2): S84–S91.

Hinchcliffe R (1994) A socio-economic factor for hearing? Journal of Audiological Medicine 3: 107–112.

Hines J (2000) Communication problems of hearing impaired patients. Nursing Standards 14(19): 33–37.

Jang Y, Mortimer JA, Haley WE, Chisolm TE, Graves AB (2002) Nonauditory determinants of self-perceived hearing problems among older adults: the role of stressful life conditions, neuroticism and social recourses. Journal of Gerontology, Medical Sciences 57A: 466–469.

Jerger J, Chmiel R, Stach B, Spretnjak M (1993) Gender affects audiometric shape in presbyacusis. Journal of the American Academy of Audiology 4: 42–49.

Joore MA, Brunenberg DEM, Chenault MN, Anteunis LJC (2003) Societal effects of hearing aid fitting among the moderately hearing impaired. International Journal of Audiology 42: 152–160.

Kampfe CM, Smith SM (1998) Intrapersonal aspects of hearing loss in persons who are older. Journal of Rehabilitation 64(2): 24–28.

Karlsson-Epsmark AK, Hansson-Scherman M (2003) Hearing confirms existence and identity – experiences from persons with presbyacusis. International Journal of Audiology 42: 106–115.

Karlsson-Espmark AK, Rosenhall U, Erlansson S, Steen B (2002) The two faces of presbyacusis: hearing impairment and psychosocial consequences. International Journal of Audiology 41: 125–135.

Keller BK, Morton JL, Thomas VS, Potter JF (1999) The effect of visual and hearing impairments on functional status. Journal of the American Geriatrics Society 47: 1319–1325.

Knutson JF, Lansing CR (1990) The relationship between communication problems and psychological difficulties in persons with profound acquired hearing loss. Journal of Speech and Hearing Disorders 55: 656–664.

Kramer SE, Kapteyn TS, Festen JM, Tobi H (1996) The relationship between self-reported hearing and measures of auditory disability. Audiology 35: 277–287.

Kramer SE, Kapteyn TS, Festen JM, Kuik DJ (1997) Assessing aspects of auditory handicap by means of pupil dilatation. Audiology 36 155–64.

Kramer SE, Kapteyn TS, Kuik DJ, Deeg DJH (2002) The association of hearing impairment and chronic diseases with psychosocial health status in older age. Journal of Aging and Health 14: 122–137.

Kricos PB (1997) Audiologic rehabilitation for the elderly: a collaborative approach. Hearing Journal 50(2): 10–19.

Kricos PB (2000) The influence of nonaudiological variables on audiological rehabilitation outcomes. Ear and Hearing 21: S7–S14.

Kricos PB, Holmes AE (1996) Efficacy of audiologic rehabilitation for older adults. Journal of the American Academy of Audiology 7: 219–229.

Lee P, Smith JP, Kington R (1999) The relationship of self-rated vision and hearing to functional status and well-being among seniors 70 years and older. American Journal of Ophthalmology 127: 447–452.

Lindenberger U, Baltes PB (1994) Sensory functioning and intelligence in old age: a strong connection. Psychology and Aging 9: 339–355.

Lubinski R, Welland RJ (1997) Normal aging and environmental effects on communication. Seminars for Speech and Language 18: 107–125.

Luey HS, Glass L, Elliott H (1995) Hard-of-hearing or deaf: issues of ears, language, culture and identity. Social Work 40: 177–187.

Lupsakko TA, Mäntyjärvi MI, Kautiainen HJ (2002) Combined functional visual and hearing impairment in a population aged 75 years and older in Finland and its influence on activities of daily living. Journal of the American Geriatrics Society 50: 1748–1749.

Marcus-Bernstein C (1986) Audiologic and nonaudiologic correlates of hearing handicap in black elderly. Journal of Speech and Hearing Research 29: 301–312.

Mulrow CD, Aguilar C, Endicott JE et al. (1990) Association between hearing impairment and the quality of life of elderly individuals. Journal of the American Geriatrics Society 38: 45–50.

Naramura H, Nakansishi N, Tatara K et al. (1999) Physical and mental correlates of hearing impairment in the elderly in Japan. Audiology 38: 24–29.

NCOA (1999). The consequences of untreated hearing loss in older persons. Research report. National Council on the Aging, Washington, DC (www.ncoa.org).

Newman C, Hug G, Jacobson GP, Sandridge S (1997) Perceived hearing handicap of patients with unilateral or mild hearing loss. Annals of Otology, Rhinology and Laryngology 106: 210–214.

Noble W (1996) What is a psychosocial approach to hearing loss? Scandinavian Audiology Supplementum 25: 6–11.

Noble W (1998) Self Assessment of Hearing and Related Functions. Whurr, London.

Noble W, Hétu R (1994) An ecological approach to disability and handicap in relation to impaired hearing. Audiology 33: 117–126.

Parving A, Biering-Sorensen M, Bech B, Christensen B, Sorensen M (1997) Hearing in the elderly > 80 years of age: prevalence of problems and sensitivity. Scandinavian Audiology 26: 99–106.

Parving A, Parving I, Erlendsson A, Christensen B (2001) Some experiences with hearing disability/handicap and quality of life measures. Audiology 40: 208–214.

Pearson JD, Morrel CH, Gordon-Salant S et al. (1995) Gender differences in a longitudinal study of age-related hearing loss. Journal of the Acoustical Society of America 97: 1196–1205.

Pichora-Fuller MK, Johnson CE, Roodenburg KEJ (1998) The discrepancy between hearing impairment and handicap in the elderly: balancing transaction and interaction. Journal of Applied Communication Research 26: 99–119.

Ramsdell DA (1947) The psychology of the hard-of-hearing and the deafened adult. In: Davis H (ed.) Hearing and Deafness. A guide for laymen. Staples Press, London, pp. 392–418.

Ringdahl A, Grimby A (2000) Severe-profound hearing impairment and health related quality of life among post-lingual deafened Swedish adults. Scandinavian Audiology 29: 266–275.

Rosenhall U, Sixt E, Sundh V, Svanborg A (1993) Correlations between presbyacusis and extrinsic noxious factors. Audiology 32: 234–243.

Rutman D, Boisseau B (1995) Acquired hearing loss: social and psychological issues in adjustment processes. International Journal of Rehabilitation Research 18: 313–323.

Salomon G, Vesterager V, Jagd M (1998) Age-related hearing difficulties. I. Hearing impairment, disability and handicap – a controlled study. Audiology 27: 164–178.

Scherer MJ, Frisina DR (1998) Characteristics associated with marginal hearing loss and subjective well-being among a sample of older adults. Journal of Rehabilitation Research and Development 35: 420–426.

Sixt E, Rosenhall U (1997) Presbyacusis related to socio-economic factors and state of health. Scandinavian Audiology 26: 133–140.

Smith SM, Kampfe CM (1997) Interpersonal relationship implications of hearing loss in persons who are older. Journal of Rehabilitation 63: 15–22.

Stephens D (1980) Evaluating the problems of the hearing impaired. Audiology 19: 205–220.

Stephens D (1996) Hearing rehabilitation in a psychosocial framework. Scandinavian Audiology 25 (suppl 43): 57–66.

Stephens D, Hétu R (1991) Impairment, disability and handicap in audiology: towards a consensus. Audiology 30: 185–200.

Stephens D, France L, Lormore K (1995) Effects of hearing impairment on the patients family and friends. Acta Otolaryngologica 115: 165–167.

Stephens D, Gianopoulos I, Kerr P (2001) Determination and classification of the problems experienced by hearing impaired elderly people. Audiology 40: 294–300.

Stephens D, Vetter N, Lewis P (2003) Investigating lifestyle factors affecting hearing aid candidature in the elderly. International Journal of Audiology 42(suppl 2): S33–S38.

Stephens SDG, Lewis PA, Charny M (1991) Assessing hearing problems within a community survey. British Journal of Audiology 25: 337–343.

Strawbridge WJ, Wallhagen MI, Schema SJ, Kaplan GA (2000) Negative consequences of hearing impairment in old age. Gerontologist 40: 320–326.

Strong CJ, Shaver JP (1991) Modifying attitudes toward persons with hearing impairments. American Annals of the Deaf 136: 252–260.

Stuck AE, Elkuch P, Dapp U et al. (2002) Feasibility and yield of a self-administered questionnaire for health risk appraisal in older people in three European countries. Age and Ageing 31: 463–467.

Tesch-Römer C (1997) Psychological effects of hearing aid use in older adults. Journal of Gerontology, Psychological Sciences 52B: 127–138.

Tesch-Römer C, Nowak M (1998) How do elderly people cope with hearing and communication problems?About the psychosocial implications of presbyacusis. (in German) Zeitschrift für Klinische Psychology 27: 105–110.

Thomas PD, Hunt WC, Garry PJ et al. (1983) Hearing acuity in a healthy elderly population: effects on emotional, cognitive and social status. Journal of Gerontology 38: 321–325.

Vesterager V, Salomon G (1991) Psychosocial aspects of hearing impairment in the elderly. Acta Otolaryngologica Supplementum 476: 215–220.

Vesterager V, Salomon G, Jagd M (1988) Age-related hearing difficulties. Audiology 27: 179–192.

Wallhagen MI (1996) 6-year impact of hearing impairment on psychosocial and physiologic functioning. Nurse Practitioner 21(9): 11–14.

Weinstein BE, Ventry IM (1982) Hearing impairment and social isolation in the elderly. Journal of Speech and Hearing Research 25: 593–599.

Werngren-Elgström M, Dehlin O, Iwarsson S (2003) Aspects of quality of life in persons with pre-lingual deafness using sign language: subjective well-being, ill-health symptoms, depression and insomnia. Archives of Gerontology and Geriatrics 37: 13–24.

WHO (2001) International Classification of Functioning, Disability and Health – ICF. World Health Organization, Geneva, Switzerland.

Wiley TL, Cruickshanks KJ, Nondahl DM, Tweed TS (2000) Self-reported hearing handicap and audiometric measures in older adults. Journal of the American Academy of Audiology 11: 67–75.

CHAPTER 8

The impact of combined vision and hearing impairment and of deafblindness

KERSTIN MÖLLER

In addition to having a hearing impairment, some people also have a reduction of their vision. The combination of auditory and visual impairments generates joint consequences that have an impact on a person's entire life situation. In this chapter, the term *deafblindness* is used to signify a functional and social condition, in which a person, due to lack of – or reduction in – seeing and hearing functions, needs (or will later need) to use touch, smell and taste, and/or to compensate cognitively (memory, conclusion, etc.) when communicating, receiving information and orienting themselves.

The purpose of this chapter is to give an account of the psychosocial effects of deafblindness in a life perspective. The chapter begins with a short description of people with deafblindness. Opinion is divided about how to define the group, and a brief account of major features characterizing this discussion is provided. A short historical presentation follows, centring on education and rehabilitation. The subsequent section on participation focuses on areas such as learning, communication, mobility, interpersonal interactions and relationships, and major life areas such as work, leisure and recreation. Environmental factors are crucial to opportunities for participation of people with deafblindness. Sounds, light and other circumstances in the environment, assistive devices, individual support and services could make possible, facilitate, impede or prevent participation by people with deafblindness. In addition to issues considered in the ICF, some further crucial matters related to deafblindness are discussed. The chapter concludes with a discussion. Issues related to the various domains are reported first for the entire group, then for people with prelingual onset of deafblindness and, finally, for those with postlingual onset.

A brief account of people with deafblindness

There are a number of genetic disorders that may cause combined reduction of vision and hearing, the most common being Usher syndrome. Moreover, during the course of life, various conditions, such as trauma, infections, viruses, drug injuries and tumours can cause loss of vision and hearing. Age-related vision and hearing impairments also occur. People with deafblindness sometimes also have additional impairments (McInnes and Treffry, 1982; Stein, Palmer and Weinberg, 1982; Fredericks and Baldwin, 1987).

The aetiologies of deafblindness in 57 pupils, 5-20 years of age in 1998/99, were compared with aetiologies in 49 pupils in 1986/87. In addition, 55 preschool children with deafness in 1998 were compared to 68 preschool children with deafness in 1988. When conducting this study, Admiraal and Huygen (2000) found several cases of unusual hereditary syndromes. Occurrences of acquired deafness – in particular congenital rubella – had decreased during the period, whereas occurrences of prenatal causes had increased. Moreover, the proportion of pupils with multiple impairments had increased from 25 to 38%. During the period 1972-79, Stein, Palmer and Weinberg (1982) studied 141 children (aged 0-16) with deafblindness and found a large proportion with additional impairments. Testing the children's hearing, they furthermore found children who could be excluded from the list of those with deafblindness.

People with deafblindness rarely have complete loss of both vision and hearing. Given the definition of deafblindness used, according to some analyses no more than 6% had both deafness and blindness: the vast majority had residual vision and/or hearing (Fredericks and Baldwin, 1987; Wolf-Schein, 1989). Among people with combined vision and hearing impairments, however, change and deterioration of remaining functions are frequent. People with combined vision and hearing impairments – i.e. deafblindness – therefore constitute a heterogeneous group (Ingraham, Daugherty and Gorrafa, 1995) which is usually subdivided according to age of onset or the main impairment.

The onset of deafblindness, before or during the development of language skills (prelingual onset), has an impact on a child's potential to develop psychologically and socially. This is often referred to as *congenital deafblindness*. Onset when language has been acquired (postlingual onset) is accompanied by altered life conditions and is usually called *acquired deafblindness*. People with onset of deafblindness in old age are usually referred to as the elderly group. Some individuals may have contextually conditioned deafblindness – depending on the function in question in combination with specific circumstances – and hence need services aimed at people with deafblindness. People with severe vision or hearing loss and people with medical diagnoses in which reduction in vision or hearing may occur, should be considered deafblindness risk groups. There are furthermore accounts of a few cases of factitious deafblindness (Miner and Feldman, 1998).

Definition of deafblindness

The concept of deafblindness does not refer to the medical terms deaf and blind, respectively, but is based on a combination of functional impairments that generate psychosocial outcomes. In the debate on how to define deafblindness, some authors stress issues related to services and education whereas others stress the degree of impairment. The situation is further complicated by the heterogeneity of the group and the way various educational systems and systems of services define their scopes of authority (McInnes and Treffry, 1982; Fredericks and Baldwin, 1987; Reed and Fontan, 1987; Wolf-Schein, 1989; Vernon and Duncan, 1990; Ingraham, Daugherty and Gorrafa, 1995; Marchant, 1996; Brennan, 1997; Aitken, 2000; Rönnberg and Borg, 2001; Bruce, 2002). In this chapter an extensive interpretation of the concept is used, relating to impairments in combination with psychosocial consequences. This understanding of the concept means including, for instance, children with Usher syndrome and elderly people with residual vision and hearing.

Historical perspective

The possibility of teaching and educating children with deafblindness seems to have been recognized for the first time by l'Abbé Deschamps, who wrote in 1779 that the first step was to give the pupils some idea of what was being pursued. He was convinced that it was possible to make pupils understand that when we want something we move our lips to ask for it. The next step was to consider how to proceed with education. In 1795 Lorenzo Hervas y Panduro outlined a method using signs of touch, smell or taste (Enerstvedt, 1996).

From the beginning of the nineteenth century there are some reports on teaching pupils with deafblindness. The pioneers and their pupils became world-famous. Some of them were associated with schools for pupils with deafness and others with schools for pupils with blindness. The idea of using fingerspelling was taken from the education of the deaf, and the idea of using letters in relief from the education of the blind (Enerstvedt, 1996).

The first special school in Sweden for pupils with deafblindness was set up in 1886. The headmistress, Elisabeth Anrep-Nordin, was a teacher with professional training in special education for the deaf. Before the school opened she travelled to the USA and Germany to study. The Swedish school was based on the assumptions that pupils with deafblindness were, firstly, good by nature and, secondly, able to learn. The school had three educational goals: to teach Christianity, to train skills necessary to perform a job and to master a language. These were similar to the goals of regular schools at that time. The educational, individualized, theoretical approach was inspired by Fröbel in Germany. Methods of language teaching were akin to methods for the deaf (Liljedahl, 1993). After the 1880 Milan conference deaf education in Sweden changed from the signing to the oral method (Eriksson, 1998). However, pupils with deafblindness were allowed to use signs – and had therefore to be kept separate from pupils with deafness, as they might otherwise exercise a bad influence. At the outset, the idea was to teach pupils to learn to talk, as they were supposed to return to their home district after school. Ragnhild Kaata, a child with deafblindness from Norway, was trained in a school for the deaf and learned to speak by holding her hand over the mouth of the speaker (Liljedahl, 1993; Enerstvedt, 1996). Handicraft, and especially weaving, had multiple purposes in the school for pupils with deafblindness in Sweden: obedience, learning a profession and keeping the hands busy to prevent low mood. A further goal of handicraft production was to obtain money for the school (Liljedahl, 1993).

The study by Liljedahl, referred to above, reveals that there are differences in early opinions about educability of pupils with deafblindness. The first school for pupils with deafblindness in Sweden was based on the assumption that pupils were educable, but Goode (1994) maintains that early opinions were that pupils with prelingual onset of deafblindness were uneducable.

Some authors describe a more recent change in the approach to people with deafblindness from the 1970s to the 1980s. While, for instance, deafblindness was earlier written and talked about as a quality of the child, now the child is referred to as a child with impairments. Such an alteration in attitudes also affects the sort of community a person with deafblindness is expected to live in. The new approach is based on the idea that children with deafblindness are expected to be together with their age peers, and adults with deafblindness are expected to live in their communities and not in protected institutional environments (Fredericks and Baldwin, 1987; Marchant, 1996). These changed attitudes have had an impact on the locations used for training activities. Earlier, training took place in special premises at institutions, but now rehabilitation increasingly takes place in natural environments, for example on the pavement going to school, in the fast-food restaurant, etc. (Gee, Harrell and Rosenberg, 1987).

In the 1960s, there were epidemics of rubella in the USA and Europe and as a result more children with deafblindness of prelingual onset were born than had ever previously been the case (Vernon and Duncan, 1990; vanDijk and Nelson, 1997). McInnes and Treffry (1982) made an important contribution to the new attitudes previously mentioned. The rubella epidemic generated a need for special education. Europeans looked for support from the USA. For example, van Dijk reported receiving support in particular from the

Perkins School for the Blind. According to van Dijk, knowledge acquired at this school was later to influence most western European countries (van Dijk and Nelson, 1997). See, further, Enerstvedt(1996) for a historical overview of education of children with deafblindness.

Activities and participation (disabilities)

Learning and applying knowledge (d1)

Deafblindness, as such, severely affects the educational context and is very demanding as far as educational, auxiliary means and attitudes are concerned whether or not the person with deafblindness has additional impairments such as intellectual disability. Pupils with deafblindness may receive special education in segregated schools or be integrated into normal schools. They may also follow general education at all levels.

Most of the spontaneous learning acquired by seeing and hearing children is disturbed by loss or substantial reduction of both distance senses. The very initial learning processes, as well as establishing relationships with parents and others, are seriously affected by prelingual onset of deafblindness (Mar and Sall, 1995; Marks, 1998). Concluding a summary of theories on van Dijk's methods concerning children with prelingual onset of deafblindness, MacFarland (1995) noted that initially this is all about relating and security, just as it is for all other children.

Communication (d3)

The point of departure in this section is the assumption that all human beings communicate, either intentionally (with or without formal language) or unintentionally. One consequence common to everyone with deafblindness is that communication is affected. Expressive communication (to express oneself) as well as – and in particular – receptive communication (to receive messages) is affected. Languages, spoken or signed, as well as communicative modalities, vary as a function of age at onset and the degree of hearing and vision losses, as well as other factors. Some people have grown up in the Deaf community and have sign language as their first language. Others have oral language as their first language (Pollard, Miner and Cioffi, 2000). The language skills of people with deafblindness range from unintentional communication to the skills of people with a university degree. Research summaries on communication with people who have deafblindness demonstrate, among other things, the heterogeneity of the group and the variety of communication methods used (Engleman, Griffin and Wheeler, 1998; Rönnberg and Borg, 2001). Communicating with people with deafblindness is very demanding in terms of the interaction partner's knowledge, skills and attitudes. However, research on communication stress on the part of the communication partners seems to be lacking.

All people with deafblindness need individualized and professional assessment of their communicative skills and appropriate individualized plans of rehabilitation, which will possibly have to be reconsidered later on in relation to altered and further reduced seeing and hearing functions (Godfrey and Costello, 1995).

Non-symbolic communication here connotes transferring messages without using symbols such as words, signs or graphics. Instead, bodily movements, facial expressions, sounds, breathing, glances, change in voice, etc. are used (Siegel-Causey and Downing, 1987). These authors deliberately do not use the expression 'prelingual communication' but rather use 'non-symbolic communication' because some people never reach the prelingual or speech level in communication.

Communication based on speech or on sign language has been very controversial as far as children with early onset of deafness are concerned, and this applies also to those children with deafness and reduced vision. Tadoma is a method where the person with deafblindness seeks to tactually feel the speech, for instance by putting a hand over the speaker's mouth or on his or her throat. The use of the Tadoma method has been evaluated (Reed et al., 1985, 1990). Use of sign language in the tactual version is dealt with, in particular, in studies by Reed et al. (1995) and Mesch (1998). Reed and colleagues have also evaluated the use of finger-spelling in the tactual version (Reed et al., 1990). Earlier it was not considered necessary for children with prelingual onset of deafblindness to learn formal signing. However, in accordance with the altered approach to deafblindness, and as these children begin to move around in the community, formal signs are increasingly introduced (van Dijk and Nelson, 1997).

Mutual glances, as a natural beginning of mutual communication and interaction between child-carer and child, will not appear in children with prelingual onset of deafblindness (Chen and Haney, 1995). There is an imminent danger that the child will go into a condition of introversion with autism-like symptoms. If communication is at an unintentional level, it is necessary to establish a mutual emotional involvement. From this point it is possible to be guided by the expressions of the person with deafblindness (Nafstad and Rödbroe, 1999). The more introverted the child or adult becomes, the more difficult it is to discover and interpret the communicative signals they send out and to respond to them in a way that they can understand (Siegel-Causey and Downing, 1987; Chen and Haney, 1995; van Dijk and Nelson, 1997; Bruce, 2003). When the child has grasped that their expression has evoked a response, intentional communication can commence (Siegel-Causey and Downing, 1987; Chen and Haney, 1995).

Several authors give accounts of intentional non-symbolic communication with people who have deafblindness. At the end of the 1970s, Goode (1994) made participant observations of two children with deafblindness and without language. He demonstrated how the children communicated in a number of ways with bodily gestures, sounds and glances. One of the children (Christina) lived in a state institution. According to Goode, at that time opinion was that children with deafblindness and intellectual disability (caused by rubella) were not educable, and hence no efforts were made to interpret the children's expressions. Goode's ambition to understand and share experiences with such a child was met with much scepticism and distrust. The other child (Bianca) lived with her parents as a much-valued member of the family. Bianca's parents made efforts to interpret her communicative expressions (stamping her foot to have some more fruit, for example) and comply with her wishes. At the same time, however, there were conflicts between Bianca's parents and her teachers because the teachers were of the opinion that Bianca could not communicate since she could not talk.

Half of the young people in Petroff's (2001) study communicated on a non-symbolic level. Most of those who used spoken language also received spoken language, and they also had a larger vocabulary than those using sign language. Petroff furthermore found a relationship between the communication method and walking. Youngsters unable to communicate using language (signed or spoken) were also unable to walk independently, whereas those with language also walked independently.

Some reports deal with difficulties in communication encountered by people with deafblindness who have a language. Sign languages are visual languages that can be adjusted and modified for users with limited peripheral vision or for tactual use (Godfrey and Costello, 1995; Mesch, 1998). Some examples of adjustments are: the speaker is at a certain distance; contrasting colours in the background and contrasting colours on speaker's/interpreter's clothing; lighting and positioning in relation to light (Cioffi, 1996). People with deafness since childhood can have poor knowledge of the language spoken and written in their country. Such shortcomings should not be confused with intellectual disability or low intelligence, but are related to the deafblindness of these people and to the kind of modified education they have (or have not) received (Godfrey and Costello, 1995; Brennan, 1997). Miner (1995) observed that it is important for children with Usher syndrome to learn sign language in its tactual version, considering these children's problem with dark adaptation, and this also applies to others with fluctuating or progressive deterioration of vision. She furthermore maintains that people with Usher syndrome may also need to use sign language in tactual version after cochlear implantation, in order both to express themselves and to receive information. Depending upon their particular background, people with deafblindness associate with either hearing or deaf subcultures. Considering the sensitivity to the issue of vision within the Deaf community, it is understandable that transition from visual to tactual sign language is made stepwise and can be traumatic (Brennan, 1997).

Godfrey and Costello (1995) give examples of communication methods for people with deafblindness who have spoken language as their first language and whose hearing is deteriorating, as is the case in Usher syndrome type 3. Miner (1997, 1999) considered the same issue in people with decreasing vision, as is the case with Usher syndrome type 2. Increasing difficulties in receiving spoken language may occur if these people previously used to combine residual hearing function with lip-reading. Godfrey and Costello point to the possibility of writing letters on the palm, perhaps in combination with using signs in tactual version, Braille, etc. (Godfrey and Costello, 1995).

It is clear that people with deafblindness sometimes use more than one modality of language and communication. In one study, 7 out of 13 people used 2 methods and 4 of them (all deaf) used both sign language and spoken language. All those making use of just one method of communication used sign language. Generally, the participants in this study reported that they had difficulties in communicating in about half of communication circumstances, and this was so in communicating about thoughts as well as feelings (Rönnberg, Samuelsson and Borg, 2002). Murdoch (1994) video-recorded interaction between children with deafblindness and one hearing and seeing partner, and observed that the partner did not always respond by using the same method as the child and also that several communication modes were used simultaneously.

Mobility (d4)

Mobility – and in particular mobility in unfamiliar surroundings – is difficult for people with deafblindness. The pathological picture of some of the syndromes generating deafblindness (for instance, Usher syndrome type 1) includes disordered balance (Kimberling and Möller, 1995). Some people with deafblindness and intellectual disability can also have mobility difficulties even in familiar settings indoors. Lancioni and Mantini (1999) described a woman with total blindness who frequently lost her orientation while moving around indoors because of her balance disorder. People in her situation may need specific technical devices and/or personal guides to find their way.

Miner (1995) described a young woman with Usher syndrome type 1, who had had a cochlear implant, having mobility training in darkness. The trainer did not understand that the woman's hearing with the cochlear implant did not give her sufficient information about the traffic situation to guarantee safe mobility. The woman felt that her fears and difficulties in crossing the street were belittled. This emphasizes the importance of instructors in mobility having knowledge of deafblindness.

In some cases people with postlingual onset of deafblindness are able to use public transport. The possibilities depend on their remaining seeing and hearing functions, their ability to absorb information from other senses (for instance, feeling the wind), their ability to orient themselves and to solve problems, and good knowledge of the language spoken around them, including the ability to express themselves in an intelligible way (Vernon and Duncan, 1990; Cioffi, 1996). In an experiment, a person with deafblindness asked for assistance, with the help of a written note, to cross a street at a street crossing. Pedestrians not offering assistance in most cases stated that they had not noticed that this person needed help (Sauerburger and Jones, 1997; Franklin and Bourquin, 2000).

The kind of medical examination required for a driver's licence is not, in all countries, sufficient to exclude people with social blindness related to decreasing peripheral vision (Tedder, 1987). People who do not know about their visual impairment (for example, in cases of late diagnosis of Usher syndrome) can find themselves involved in traffic accidents when driving (Hicks, 1978). Tedder (1987) points out the need to counsel young people and adults on responsible attitudes to driving in relation to their reduced vision. Giving up driving is one of the most difficult experiences for a person with deafblindness. When they have to stop driving, further consequences are triggered off within all life areas, not only those related to transportation, and stress and grief can result (Brennan, 1997).

Domestic life (d6)

In the 1970s, the general position in the USA and Europe was that people with deafblindness should be cared for in institutions. Now, their life is normalized to an increasing extent and they live in less sheltered environments: with parents or independently. No studies dealing with housing etc. for people with postlingual onset of deafblindness have been found. Research in progress, as well as personal contacts with people with postlingual onset of deafblindness in a number of European countries and in other parts of the world, indicates that these people usually live in their own homes and are (or have been) working. Sometimes they also have a family and children, with or without deafblindness.

In a study by Pteroff (2001) more than half of the youngsters lived with their parents and just a few lived independently. Various studies indicate that parents of children with prelingual onset of deafblindness do not think that their child will live independently in the future (Wolf-Schein, 1989; Petroff,

2001). Moreover, parents of children or young people with postlingual onset of deafblindness, for instance with Usher syndrome, vary in their opinion about whether their children could manage a household by themselves (Miner, 1995).

From a gender perspective, difficulties in independently managing household tasks, such as cooking and cleaning, might be a worse loss for a woman than for a man. If so, such practical barriers have an emotional significance similar to that of being no longer able to drive (Miner, 1995).

Interpersonal interactions and relationships (d7)

Common to all people with deafblindness is the fact that problems of communication make interpersonal interactions more difficult, particularly for people with prelingual onset of deafblindness.

Mar and Sall (1995) conducted intervention research, focusing on three children with deafblindness. The aim was to examine the children's engagement in social activities with their age peers without impairments, with the purpose of implementing improvements. Two of the children had intellectual disability in addition to deafblindness and communicated intentionally on a non-symbolic level (gestures, facial expressions, etc.). The third child expressed himself through spoken language and could also receive speech with the help of a hearing aid and an FM system. Initially the study found that the children – including the child with spoken language – had relatively few friends. Any friends were as a rule associated with specific situations, such as the church or the immediate neighbourhood. The child with speech, who was in a regular class at the local school, did not have adequate social contacts at school either. During the course of the study, the children's interaction with their age peers and new acquaintances increased but it was not possible to decide whether this was due to the intervention or other circumstances. Petroff (2001) also indicated occurrence of social isolation among young people with deafblindness.

One study of siblings' interactions with their brothers and sisters with deafblindness indicated unequal roles, with the child without deafblindness frequently taking a supporting role. The more difficulties siblings had in communicating with each other, the more joint activities were negatively affected. Many siblings did not play with the brother or sister with deafblindness, or even avoided them. When playing games with friends, more than half of the siblings did not include their brother or sister with deafblindness in these activities. Nor did siblings adjust their behaviour by, for instance, providing information about things going on in the surroundings or during transportation. Seeing and hearing siblings were furthermore usually self-taught about ways of communicating with their sibling with deafblindness.

They also expressed wishes to meet other children who had siblings with deafblindness. Writers stress the need of further research into this area and the need for information and training of siblings by professionals, in particular support to improve communication with their siblings with deafblindness (Heller et al., 1999).

Regarding postlingual onset of deafblindness, there are contradictory reports about interaction within the family. There are some reports about families with children with Usher syndrome, for example, where parents learn sign language (Torrie, 1978; Miner, 1995), but there are also reports of parents who can barely or not at all communicate with their children (Miner, 1995; Brennan, 1997). Young people and adults with Usher syndrome may encounter increasing difficulties in reading their parent's lips when their vision deteriorates and, if the parents do not know sign language, communication is made more difficult (Miner, 1995).

Relationships between children or young people with Usher syndrome and their age peers may be affected by decreasing peripheral vision, associated with Usher syndrome, when a person with deafblindness does not notice that another person has opened a conversation. The person with deafblindness could then be thought of as rude or stupid and could even be abused (Vernon and Duncan, 1990; Miner, 1995). Pupils with deafblindness are reported to be socially isolated from age peers when integrated into regular schools and also when attending special schools (Ingraham, Daugherty and Gorrafa, 1995; Miner, 1995). Attention has also been paid to matters concerning information, training skills and giving support to age peers of young people with deafblindness (Brennan, 1997; Goetz and O'Farrell, 1999). Social interaction for pupils with deafblindness can be improved through powerful support and information to their peers (Mar and Sall, 1995).

People with Usher syndrome (types 1 and 2) have reported that friends withdrew when their seeing functions deteriorated (Miner, 1997, 1999).

A number of researchers stress the importance of creating opportunities for people with deafblindness to meet with others who also have deafblindness (Hammer, 1978; Fillman, Leguire and Sheridan, 1989; Vernon and Duncan, 1990; Miner, 1995; Brennan, 1997).

Miner (1995) gives accounts of difficulties encountered by seeing and hearing children when parents have Usher syndrome type 1. The children have felt the responsibility of interpreting for their parent(s) to be too much for their age (Miner, 1995).

Tedder (1987) maintains that there are risks of physical and psychological violence as well as broken relationships, but the research examined in this chapter provided no information about incidents of violence.

Major life areas (d8)

Education (d810)

Petroff (2001) conducted a survey in the USA, directed at parents of young people (aged 18–24) with deafblindness who left school in 1996. The youngsters' last educational placement had been segregated special education In this study half of the pupils had left school because they had reached the maximum age and barely half had graduated with a diploma. After leaving school more than half of the pupils were still illiterate. Miner (1997) maintains that pupils with Usher syndrome type 2, and having hearing loss, either attend special schools for pupils with deafness or are integrated into regular local schools.

A number of studies have demonstrated that pupils with deafblindness do not always have access to specially trained teachers, and also how such circumstances affect the pupils' possibilities of learning (Ingraham, Daugherty and Gorrafa, 1995; Kirchner and Diament, 1999a; Bruce, 2002). Ingraham and colleagues give an example of how substantial support can be provided for pupils with deafblindness, guided by pupils' present and future needs. Cooperation between various authorities, as well as flexible solutions to financing support services, were required and implemented. Teachers needed to prepare lessons several days in advance, as the lessons had to be interpreted and educational material had to be written out in Braille, for instance. Special resource teachers played important roles in developing education. Authors repeatedly stress the importance of considering the specific needs of each and every pupil. The pupils referred to in this example were subsequently moved from special school settings to their local general school. When considering educational placement, issues regarding risks of isolation also have to be taken into account (Ingraham, Daugherty and Gorrafa, 1995).

In Petroff's study (2001), 17% of pupils had received post-secondary education but none of them attended a 4-year college. Participants were provided with trained deafblind counsellors at school. Other studies report people with deafblindness having post-secondary and university education (Enerstvedt, 1996; Rönnberg, Samuelsson and Borg, 2002).

As a result of their deafblindness, many young people and adults have inadequate all-round education and therefore lack knowledge of, for instance, matters related to sexuality. Even people who have acquired deafblindness later in life, and people who have been married and have brought up children, can need special adult education. The Helen Keller National Center in the USA provides an example of tailored sexual education. Information is provided in spoken language, in sign language and also in written form using the most appropriate means: for instance Braille, photographs, large letters. Models of female and male anatomy are used to name parts of the body, to prepare for gynaecological examination and to provide information about instruments and procedures that will be used during examination, as well as information about safe sex and contraceptive counselling. The education could also deal with masturbation methods, and information on when and where masturbation is appropriate. Students are also informed about parts of the body that are appropriate or not appropriate for touching. If they need help with hygiene and personal care, they are informed about circumstances when it may be right for assistants and inter-preters to give tactile support, and when not. Information on relational issues and pregnancy is also included. The authors emphasize that sexual education of people with deafblindness must be viewed in a life perspective and be provided throughout the course of the person's life (Ingraham et al., 2000).

Work (d840)

Matters regarding the labour market and vocational training are rarely dealt with. Research into the occurrence of employment among adults with deafblindness, the kind of jobs they have, experiences of work, relations to workmates, etc. is still lacking.

As with the issue of housing, parents of youngsters with deafblindness seem not to believe that their children will be able to manage a job (Wolf-Schein, 1989; Petroff, 2001).

One study of supported employment demonstrates how work prefer-ences can be tested and considered before choosing work tasks and work placement for a person with prelingual onset of deafblindness and without language (Parsons et al., 1998). Petroff (2001) writes that only 8% of the young people in his study were reported to have had vocational training in competitive or supported work settings as part of their secondary education. In general, long-term vocational rehabilitation, adjustment of the workplace, technical devices, etc. are important preconditions for the prospective employment (Vernon and Duncan, 1990; Miner, 1995; Petroff, 2001). Bourquin, Mascia and Rusenski (2002) examined a service programme for adults with postlingual onset of deafblindness aiming at employment. The quantity and quality of services delivered were usually dependent upon issues that were not related to the vocational rehabilitation process as such, but rather to matters such as transport to and from any future workplace which frequently impeded success. Marchant (1996) gave an account of another kind of workplace-related support: workmates of a man with deafblindness were given information about deafblindness and were taught sign language, and subsequently accepted the man.

In spite of various measures to promote employment, most people with deafblindness are unemployed: more than 80% of the participants in Petroff's (2001) study.

For people with postlingual onset of deafblindness, it is imperative to obtain an accurate diagnosis as soon as possible. Vocational counselling and choice of profession are important (Davenport et al., 1978), and also complicate matters because of difficulties in making prognoses about when and how rapidly vision and/or hearing will deteriorate (Miner, 1995). There are cases of people with Usher syndrome who have invested much time and money in vocational training, which they later had to abandon when their vision deteriorated. They had not been informed about their diagnosis or prognosis (Hicks, 1978). Vernon (1969) mentions that many people with Usher syndrome are forced to stop working before retirement age because of progressive visual impairment. There has been no research focusing on the labour market experiences of people with postlingual onset of deafblindness and hence we do not know much about this.

Leisure and recreation (d920)

Access to leisure-time activities for people with deafblindness can be dependent on services (for instance, guides or transportation), as well as the skills of the specific person. Several studies deal with the importance of physical activities and the limited opportunities for people with deafblindness to engage in such sports as bowling, swimming, walks, etc. (Hammer, 1978; Vernon and Duncan, 1990; Petroff, 2001). Children with deafblindness were included in one study dealing with physical activities and fitness of children with visual impairments, and findings were then compared to those of children without visual impairments. Children with a double impairment were significantly worse off (Liberman and Hugh, 2001).

The most frequent leisure-time activities in a study of adults with postlingual onset of deafblindness were walking, swimming, computer work and reading. Even if most of them participated in some activity, 60% were not satisfied with their current level of participation in recreational activities. They wanted, for instance, social activities, activities requiring good physical shape, dancing and boat trips (Liberman and Stuart, 2002). The low level of participation was due to lack of transportation, co-participants, suitable programmes, guides or time, and to negative attitudes (Reed and Fontan, 1987; Petroff, 2001; Liberman and Stuart, 2002).

People with Usher syndrome and similar visual impairments encounter specific problems because of their decreasing peripheral visual field, light sensitivity and contrast sensitivity (Miner, 1995). Engagement in associations where speakers make use of sign language can also cause problems: people with decreased peripheral vision may have difficulty in tracking the shifting turns of speakers, and can therefore find themselves becoming outsiders (Miner, 1995). Furthermore, they may withdraw from evening activities because of difficulties with dark adaptation (Vernon and Duncan, 1990).

Environmental factors

Environmental factors can facilitate as well as act as barriers for people with deafblindness.

Products and technology (e1)

Technical devices – in addition to hearing aids, FM systems and cochlear implantation to compensate for hearing impairments, and glasses and a white stick in the case of visual impairments – can provide assistance for people with deafblindness. Assistive devices specific to deafblindness and unusual devices are at the centre of the following discussion.

Research and development of vibratory devices to facilitate perception are in progress (Borg, 1997; Borg, Neovius and Kjellander, 2001; Borg, Rönnberg and Neovius, 2001). These devices have also been used to facilitate indoor mobility (Lancioni and Mantini, 1999). When deafblind subjects were asked to rank assistive devices, optical and vibrotactile signals were the most preferred (Rönnberg, Samuelsson and Borg, 2002).

An auxiliary means of independent mobility is the use of guide dogs specially trained for people with deafblindness. Dogs can also be trained to pay attention to and localize sounds. However, 'hearing dogs' cannot be used for mobility and vice versa (Vernon and Duncan, 1990).

An example of low-tech assistive equipment is the use of photographs. Books with photographs of a pupil's everyday surroundings and of motivating events – favourite activities such as playing in the pool – have been used for interactive exchange (Goetz and O'Farrell, 1999).

For people with deafblindness who know how to write, textphone (stationary) and Tellatuch are useful devices. Tellatuch is a small portable apparatus on which messages to a person with deafblindness are written using a keyboard while the receiver reads messages in Braille (Vernon and Duncan, 1990). IT has provided possibilities of obtaining information through the internet and making contact by e-mail, all of which is a new research field, not yet entered (Miner, 1999).

Assistive devices are useful only when they work. Devices that are difficult to use, or broken or otherwise non-functional, can have disastrous consequences, as has been demonstrated in a study of pupils (Giangreco, Edelman and Nelson, 1998).

Natural environment and human-made changes to environment (e2)

In several causes of deafblindness, for instance Usher syndrome, seeing functions alter when light conditions change; for instance, dazzle from snow or bright sunshine, haze, mist, dusk and darkness can cause problems. The use of ultraviolet filters cannot fully compensate for such changes in the environment. Sensitivity to contrasts and light can make a green board with white chalk most difficult to perceive, and a white board can be dazzling (Fillman, Leguire and Sheridan, 1989).

Support and relationships (e3)

Research dealing with support and relationships is included in the earlier section on 'Interpersonal interactions and relationships'. Here, the question of professional support is considered.

Some authors have demonstrated the positive impact of interveners (a kind of personal assistant). Programmes with interveners for children as well as adults with prelingual onset of deafblindness have been evaluated. Progress was reported for people with deafblindness, and their parents also viewed the measure in a positive way (Watkins et al., 1994; Hammer and Carlsson, 1996).

Some reports deal with the significance of interpreters and the specific requirements for interpreters interpreting for people with deafblindness as compared to interpreting between spoken language and sign language for people with deafness (Petronio, 1988; Bourquin, 1996). People with deafblindness have specific needs that vary from person to person and sometimes between various settings of interpretation. When interpreting for people with deafblindness, the interpreter has to be flexible and aware of a number of conditions that have to be taken into consideration (Petronio, 1988). Even if interpretation is visual, the scope of signs and also the particular signs used have to be adjusted and the interpretation has to be supplemented with information about events and objects in the environment, etc. (Petronio, 1988).

Attitudes (e4)

Unlike people with hearing impairments, people with deafness who are members of the Deaf community usually do not view their deafness as a disability but rather as part of their identity and a source of pride and support (Miner, 1995, 1997). Visual impairments are, however, particularly traumatic to people with deafness because of the importance of vision for their communication and perception. Moreover, as Cioffi (1996) puts it, there is an almost phobic fear of blindness in the Deaf community. Young people in the Deaf community may deny any visual impairment and the need for specific adaptations due to loss of vision, use of white stick, mobility training, etc. (Miner, 1995; Cioffi, 1996).

There are contradictory reports on relationships and interaction between people with deafblindness and people with only deafness. Brennan (1997) maintains that, even though most people with deafness know someone with deafblindness, they usually have no patience with people who use tactual sign language. Vernon and Duncan (1990), on the other hand, point out that people with deafness easily understand the kind of problems that light sensitivity generates for those with Usher syndrome and can be supportive if they are informed in advance.

Given that deafblindness is relatively rare, most professionals may not have much knowledge of it, or about how to use sign language. Frequently professionals turn to parents or the guide and not to the person with deafblindness. If the parents do not know sign language, the chances are that the person with deafblindness is treated like a child and people talk above her or his head (Miner, 1995). Well-educated people, people with high professional positions, parents and others who have deafblindness report experiences of other people looking down on them or patronizing them (Miner, 1995).

Services, systems and policies (e5)

People with deafblindness are to a large extent dependent upon services and support in order to live an active and participating life. The present literature review reveals considerable inadequacies in these respects.

Petroff's (2001) study reports on services received by young people during their last year at school. Only 60% had received speech and language services – a low number considering that a large proportion of the youngsters did not communicate using formal language. Only about 30% had received orientation and mobility services, even though about 50% of the youngsters in the group under study moved around on their own.

As far as preparations for adult life are concerned, 40% of the young people in Petroff's (2001) study lacked a written, individual plan of transition and almost a quarter had none whatsoever.

Several authors report insufficient coordination of services; moreover, people who supplied services lacked knowledge about deafblindness (Wolf-Schein, 1989; Goode, 1994; Miner, 1995, 1997; Giangreco et al., 1999; Kirchner and Diament, 1999b; Petroff, 2001; Bourquin, Mascia and Rusenski, 2002; Janssen, Riksen-Walraven and van Dijk, 2002). Giangreco (2000) summarizes various methods of providing services. Some reports point out problems with large staff turnover and burnout symptoms among those professionals working closest to people with deafblindness. In a 4-year project, comprising 358 professionals working with 18 pupils with deafblindness, only 29 remained for the entire project and, of these, 10 did not come into contact with the pupil more than about once a month (Giangreco et al., 1999) Giangreco and colleagues also point out risks of conflict between specially trained personnel and, for instance, teachers of children integrated into regular schools (Goode, 1994; Giangreco, Edelman and Nelson, 1998).

Personal factors

Psychological and mental conditions

Murdoch found several difficulties in testing the mental development of children with deafblindness: the instruments assumed that the child could either hear or see (Murdoch, 1994).

For people with prelingual onset of deafblindness, there are some 25 reports about behavioural disorders such as repetitive habits (swinging the body, bringing fingers in front of eyes), self-injury (biting or scratching oneself), aggressive behaviour towards others (scratching, biting, pinching) and – common to most people with deafblindness – introversion (Tweedie, 1974; Yarnall and Dodginson-Ensor, 1980; Rapoff, Altman and Christopherson-Edward, 1980; McInnes and Treffry, 1982; Fewell and Rich, 1987; Fredericks and Baldwin, 1987; Lancioni et al., 1991; Myrbakk, 1991; Peine et al., 1991; Romer and Schoenberg, 1991; Luiselli, 1992; Sisson, Hersen and Van-Hasselt, 1993; Goode, 1994; Watkins et al., 1994; Chen and Haney, 1995; van Dijk and Nelson, 1997; Nafstad and Rödbroe, 1999, to mention only some). It is easy to be misled and believe that behavioural disorders are associated with prelingual onset of deafblindness. However, most of the research focuses on just one or a few cases of behavioural disorders and does not provide information about prevalence. In Petroff's (2001) study, about half of the youngsters were reported to have problematic or challenging behaviour.

There are also many reports about measures to reduce or halt behavioural disorders. Such measures include throwing water on the child (Peine et al., 1991), smells (Rapoff, Altman and Christopherson-Edward, 1980; Gross, 1994), tastes (McDaniel, Kocim and Barton, 1984), technical devices (Lancioni et al., 1991), positive reinforcement and encouragement (Yarnall, 1980; Luiselli and Lolli, 1987; Luiselli, 1988; Myrbakk, 1991; Sisson, Hersen and Van-Hasselt, 1993) and medication (Luiselli, 1991).

Some studies, concentrating on environmental factors, point out that certain treatments generate stress in children with prelingual onset of deafblindness. If the stress is not removed, behavioural disorders will result (Tweedie, 1974; McInnes and Treffry, 1982; van Dijk and Nelson, 1997). Misunderstandings or abortive efforts to communicate could lead to frustration and trigger off aggressive or self-injuring behaviour (Janssen, Riksen-Walraven and van Dijk, 2002). Other studies indicate that behavioural disorders can decrease or cease as a result of changes in the behaviour of seeing and hearing adults (van Dijk and Nelson, 1997; Marks, 1998; Janssen, Riksen-Walraven and van Dijk, 2002, 2003).

There are some studies dealing with psychological issues relating to the postlingual onset of deafblindness. Vernon and Hammer (1996) argue that various measures and tests in the field of psychology are not suitable for people with deafblindness. The difficulties of communication caused by deafblindness are not related to a person's mental capacity.

There are different opinions on psychiatric illness as a common complication in the case of people with Usher syndrome. There are reports of psychological complications in cases of Usher syndrome, but there is no proof of increased levels of psychiatric complications (Kimberling and Möller, 1995). There are reports of depression, psychosis and suicidal tendencies as elements of an existential crisis for people losing vision and hearing (Miner, 1995, 1996, 1997; Vernon and Hammer, 1996; Hess-Rover et al., 1999). Vernon and Duncan (1990), moreover, maintain that elderly people with deafblindness can develop additional impairments, such as depression and dementia.

Emotional consequences

Deafblindness is a highly emotional topic. This is evident from the literature as well as from personal experiences. People with deafblindness, their relatives and professionals all express strong emotions such as grief, guilt, shame, anger and frustration – more or less observably so in the accounts given previously in this chapter.

People with Usher syndrome express emotions relating to loss of independence when their vision deteriorates in a number of ways (Hicks, 1978; Miner, 1995, 1997, 1999). The inadequate behaviour of people with Usher syndrome, such as refusal to use a white stick, guide dog or guide – in spite of obvious needs and these things having been prescribed for them – could be related to denial. Acting-out and promiscuity could, in fact, be about a refusal to deal with grief and pain (Fillman, Leguire and Sheridan, 1989; Vernon and Duncan, 1990). Hammer (1978) argued that people with Usher syndrome who do not demonstrate stress are possibly out of touch with reality. He maintains that attention should be paid to this group. Rönnberg, Samuelsson and Borg (2002) found emotional problems in a group of adults with deafblindness. A positive correlation was found between the inability to discover and localize people and events in the surroundings on the one hand, and pessimistic thoughts on the other.

Frequent feelings of loss and grief are common to people with Usher syndrome, as a result of successive changes in seeing and hearing functions (Miner, 1995, 1997, 1999). In addition, practical consequences, such as reduction of independence, loss of driver's licence or the introduction of a white stick, are emotionally loaded (Brennan, 1997; Miner, 1995, 1997). The ongoing loss brings up past losses that need to be re-examined and reworked, so there is a need for recurrent psychological support and therapy (Miner, 1999). Miner, as well as Vernon and Hammer (1996), points out the need for therapy in the language and mode suitable to the person with deafblindness. Miner, in particular, stresses the importance of therapists having skills and personal strength to handle their own anxiety. This can be crucial in the case of therapists who themselves have deafness, as they cherish their own vision and fear losing it.

Parents of children with prelingual onset of deafblindness can have strong emotions, such as frustration, due to feeble and hard-to-interpret responses from the children during interaction (Chen and Haney, 1995). Grief and feelings of guilt among parents of children with Usher syndrome are also reported (Torrie, 1978; Fillman, Leguire and Sheridan, 1989; Miner, 1995, 1997). Families of a person with Usher syndrome can need support in talking to each other about their emotions relating to the syndrome (Miner, 1999). The previously mentioned reports of elevated staff turnover furthermore indicate that the care of people with deafblindness is stressful for health-care professionals too (Goode, 1994; Giangreco et al., 1999).

Other social effects

This section deals with issues not included in the previous accounts linked to the ICF that are particularly relevant when deafblindness is considered: chains of consequences, impact on psychology, importance of knowledge about deafblindness, public health matters, emotional consequences, genetic issues and alternative strategies.

Chains of consequences

Characteristically, the consequences of deafblindness are linked in long chains. For example, combined vision and hearing impairment affects communication, which in turn affects relationships with other people, which then causes social isolation. Each link in the chain contributes to further consequences at the same time as it is connected to and dependent upon earlier links. Taken together, chains of consequences generate an impact on life that reaches far beyond any sum of single consequences. A number of references provide examples of outcomes generated by previous consequences.

Children with prelingual onset of deafblindness run the risk of acquiring persistent learned helplessness. According to Marks (1998), learned helplessness emerges when a person cannot control their surroundings or the results of their actions. The risk is that teachers and caregivers foster a dependency by expecting too little from a child.

Miner (1995) described how an elderly woman with Usher syndrome type 1 fell down in the street when she was out walking alone. Hitherto the woman had usually been escorted by a relative and, by the time of the event described, she had not yet learnt to use a white stick. Several people passing by rushed to help her, but her vision was not sufficient to read their lips and they could not use sign language.

Further examples of chains of consequences are presented in studies of people with postlingual onset of deafblindness (Fillman, Leguire and Sheridan, 1989; Vernon and Duncan, 1990; Miner, 1995, 1997; Cioffi, 1996; Brennan, 1997).

Knowledge about deafblindness – other people's skills

In quite a few references, the knowledge and skills of parents, relatives and professionals are pointed out as being crucial for positive development among people with deafblindness. From the accounts given previously, it is obvious that specific knowledge is needed from the very initial interactions with children with prelingual onset of deafblindness. This is pointed out in a number of studies (Chen and Haney, 1995; Nafstad and Rödbroe, 1999; Bruce, 2002, 2003).

However, there is no research regarding, for instance, the early impact of seeing functions on playing games and education. Furthermore, studies of the scope of knowledge about these issues among educationalists, parents and others coming into contact with children with postlingual onset of deafblindness, for example children with Usher syndrome, are also lacking.

There is rarely specific accommodation for people with deafblindness, and those who need to live in some kind of sheltered accommodation frequently do so within programmes directed to people with other impairments. If personnel and other residents cannot communicate in a manner receivable to the person with deafblindness, he or she becomes more and more isolated (Vernon and Duncan, 1990).

Public health issues and health threats

There are specific health threats related to deafblindness. Besides the risk of traffic accidents or of being the victim of criminals (Cioffi, 1996), there are also threats related to lack of information on public health matters, such as food recommendations, warnings concerning use of tobacco and alcohol, warning notes on medicines and so on. No attention has been paid to deafblindness from a public health perspective in the reviewed literature.

Health threats related to labour are noticed in one study, which in addition points out that occupations traditionally regarded as dangerous are not necessarily dangerous to people with deafblindness. It is rather their occupational skills and adjustment to deafblindness that are decisive (Vernon and Duncan, 1990).

Genetics-related issues

Psychosocial aspects of genetically caused deafblindness are dealt with in a few studies, in all cases in relation to Usher syndrome

Even though Usher syndrome is genetically caused, most children with Usher syndrome are born to seeing and hearing parents. Initially, parents are informed that their child is born with deafness; not until later do they learn that the child also has a serious and progressive visual impairment. This can cause a crisis for the parents, and relational problems associated with the child can emerge. Parents need to learn sign language and to meet other parents in similar situations, as well as children and adults with Usher syndrome, to gain experience (Miner, 1995). Miner's observations show that rehabilitation in the area of deafblindness needs to encompass not only the person with impairments but also parents, siblings and other family members as well as personnel and officials, as specific knowledge and conduct are required.

Because Usher syndrome is genetically caused, parents as well as the person with Usher syndrome have feelings of guilt, according to Miner (1995, 1997). She also notes that family members cannot always talk to each other about these feelings. There are people who do not find out that they have Usher syndrome until they are adults (at 25, 35 or 40 years of age), although their parents have known this for years. Miner maintains that children with genetically caused syndromes should be informed as soon as the diagnosis is decided, claiming support for this opinion from several studies. Explanations should furthermore be provided that are suited to the child's cognitive and mental level of development, and questions should be answered in an honest way (Tedder, 1987; Miner, 1995).

Not everyone with Usher syndrome tells their children and grandchildren that they have a genetically hereditary disease and that descendants could be carriers of the defective gene (Miner, 1995). Some people who know that they have Usher syndrome marry and have children early on, whereas others choose not to have children. Harrod (1978) maintained that families that receive genetic information about Usher syndrome must be encouraged to assimilate the facts. Considering such information, they are, according to Harrod, able to judge alternatives and make their own informed choices regarding children. Harrod maintains that no decision is incorrect as long as it is based on information. In previous contacts with people with postlingual onset of deafblindness, I have learned that some people have experienced abusive treatment by physicians, forbidding them to have children because of their heredity.

Alternative strategies and skills

In order to compensate for deafblindness, it may be necessary to develop alternative strategies, for instance various methods of making use of smell, taste, sensitivity of the skin, memory or ability to draw conclusions. Such consequences of deafblindness have not been considered in the literature. However, Goode (1994, p. 17) has taken an interest in alternative strategies and provides some interesting observations. Moreover, he maintains that:

> Establishing an understanding (intersubjectivity) with the children in their 'own terms' would be significant not only for our understanding of them but for our efforts at teaching and socializing.

Goode (1974) described a situation during the previously mentioned participant observation. He was going to feed one of the children with deafblindness but did not succeed in holding the spoon in the right position. The child then took his hand with her hand and brought it to the right position. In other words the child, who was considered uneducable, was able to correct him. Goode maintained that she understood routines and could teach them as well. The same child used her mouth to explore her surroundings and Goode gave an account of how she wetted things she wanted to know more about with her saliva. He also described something he calls *esoteric communication*, in which knowledge is transmitted from the person with deafblindness although the receiver cannot explain how this was done. There is also a feeling that the child has known about events before they occur. Such communication cannot be explained scientifically.

People with decreasing peripheral vision can compensate by turning their heads more often without being themselves aware that they do something different from other people (Vernon and Duncan, 1990).

Discussion

The present overview demonstrates that, on the whole, our knowledge of the psychosocial consequences of deafblindness is fragmentary. Basically, questions about the way people with deafblindness live their lives – in particular adults and elderly people – remain unanswered. By and large the reviewed literature is prescriptive rather than descriptive, and does not search for causes. Also, it chiefly relates to children with prelingual onset of deafblindness. Services offered to people with deafblindness follow the same pattern, according to Pollard, Miner and Cioffi (2000).

Few studies are based upon empirical information gathered for scientific purposes. This overview is based exclusively upon references found in scientific databases. In addition to such references, there is a number of more or less scientific reports emanating from conferences and projects.

However, the overview illustrates that the consequences of deafblindness are decisive to the way that life can be lived. Furthermore, the consequences of deafblindness affect not only the person with the impairment, but also their family and other people in their surroundings. Environmental factors play a decisive role when it comes to activities and participation, and sometimes even with regard to the impairment itself (for instance, darkness causing a temporary deterioration in the vision of people with Usher syndrome, or inadequate rehabilitation of those with prelingual onset of deafblindness causing stress and generating behavioural disorders). It has also been shown that specific measures by trained professionals are required to achieve optimal living conditions. However, one report after another reveals that – particularly in cases of prelingual onset of deafblindness – rehabilitation, education and services are insufficient and generate activity limitations and participation restrictions, adding further threats to health.

The psychosocial consequences of deafblindness with onset during old age is not considered in the literature reviewed here. Indeed, elderly people are included in a few studies but attention has not been paid to issues related to old age (Wolf-Schein, 1989; Vernon and Duncan, 1990; Miner, 1995; Rönnberg and Borg, 2001; Liberman and Stuart, 2002; Rönnberg, Samuelsson and Borg, 2002). However, there are a number of reports originating from conferences and projects, specifically dealing with the situation of older people with deafblindness in Norway (Statens sentralteam, 1999), the Netherlands (Stoop, 1996) and the UK (Greaves, 1999).

There is an urgent need for research into the social consequences of deafblindness, particularly various conditions of children and young people with postlingual onset of deafblindness and consequences of deafblindness for adults and elderly people. The few references available concerning adults, such as the studies reported by Petroff (2001) and Miner (1995, 1997), with few exceptions, lack accounts of the relationship between the degree of visual and hearing impairments on the one hand and the psychosocial conditions on the other.

At present, a longitudinal project (5 years) is in progress in the Nordic countries, dealing with the social consequences where alterations in communication are required as a result of deteriorating sight and hearing. This project – which has not generated any scientific papers so far – is an example of much-needed research. Furthermore, research into the emergence and impact of disability movements in the case of people with deafblindness is non-existent.

Another unexplored area is the use of alternative strategies. Instead of focusing on problems associated with deafblindness, we could look upon people with deafblindness as survivors with unique talents. Associations created by people with deafblindness and emerging deafblind communities are other fields that could be investigated in the future. In our capacity as human beings with vision as well as hearing, we can learn from people with deafblindness if we make the effort to perceive the world as it presents itself to them. A quote from Goode, relating to Christina – a child with prelingual onset of deafblindness in his study – illustrates the importance of a universalistic view when researching about and with people with deafblindness. Goode points out sources of joy and belonging in spite of barriers caused by lack of a common spoken language:

> If we can accept and understand the malleability and heterogeneity involved in the expressions of these basic projects in the life world, then we can stop one of our central self-deceptions and move away from a view of humankind that raises us above other creatures or that affirms one 'kind' of human as better than another. Chris and I may have had our 'differences', but these were differences of degree, not of quality. This is probably the most important ethical lesson I learnt from Christina (Goode, 1994, p. 42).

References

Admiraal RJC, Huygen PLM (2000) Changes in the aetiology of hearing impairment in deaf-blind pupils and deaf infant pupils at an institute for the deaf. International Journal of Pediatric Otorhinolaryngology 55: 133–142.

Aitken S (2000) Understanding deafblindness. In: Aitken S, Buultjens M, Clark C, Eyre JI, Pease L (eds) Teaching Children who are Deafblind Contact Communication and Learning. David Fulton, London.

Borg E (1997) Cutaneous senses for detection and localization of environmental sound sources: a review and tutorial. Scandinavian Audiology 26: 195–206.

Borg E, Neovius L, Kjellander M (2001) A three-microphone system for real-time directional analysis: Toward a device for environmental monitoring in deaf-blind. Journal of Rehabilitation Research and Development 38: 265–272.

Borg E, Rönnberg J, Neovius L (2001) Vibratory-coded directional analysis: Evaluation of a three- microphone/four-vibrator DSP system. Journal of Rehabilitation Research and Development 38: 257–263.

Bourquin E, Mascia J, Rusenski S (2002) Community-based service for deaf-blind consumers: a successful rehabilitation and vocational model. Journal of Visual Impairment and Blindness 96: 668–671.

Bourquin EA (1996) Using interpreters with deaf-blind clients: What professional service providers should know. Rehabilitation and Education for Blindness and Visual Impairment 27: 149–154.

Brennan M (1997) Point of view mental health issues of deaf-blind adults. Journal of the American Deafness and Rehabilitation Association 30: 28–35.

Bruce SM (2002) Impact of a communication intervention model on teachers' practice with children who are congenitally deaf-blind. Journal of Visual Impairment and Blindness 96: 154–168.

Bruce SM (2003) The importance of shared communication forms. Journal of Visual Impairment and Blindness 97: 106–109.

Chen D, Haney M (1995) An early intervention model for infants who are deaf-blind. Journal of Visual Impairment and Blindness 89: 213–221.

Cioffi J (1996) Orientation and mobility and the Usher syndrome client. Journal of Vocational Rehabilitation 6: 175–183.

Davenport SLH, O'Nuallain S, Omenn GS, Wilkus RJ (1978) Usher syndrome in four hard-of-hearing siblings. Pediatrics 62: 578–583.

Dijk J van, Nelson C (1997) History and change in the education of children who are deaf-blind since the rubella epidemic of the 1960s: Influence of methods developed in the Netherlands. Deafblind Perspectives 5: 1–5.

Enerstvedt RT (1996) Legacy of the Past. Those who are gone but have not left. Nord-Press, Dronninglund.

Engleman MD, Griffin HC, Wheeler L (1998) Deaf-blindness and communication: practical jnowledge and strategies. Journal of Visual Impairment and Blindness 92: 783–798.

Eriksson P (1998) The History of Deaf People. Daufr, Örebro.

Fewell RR, Rich JS (1987) Reducing severe behavior problems among persons with dual sensory impairments: An evaluation of a technical assistance model. Journal of the Association for Persons with Severe Handicaps 12: 2–10.

Fillman R, Leguire LE, Sheridan M (1989) Consideration for serving adolescents with Usher's syndrome. Rehabilitation and Education for Blindness and Visual Impairment 21: 19–25.

Franklin P, Bourquin E (2000) Picture this: A pilot study for improving street crossing for deaf-blind travelers. Rehabilitation and Education for Blindness and Visual Impairment 31: 173–179.

Fredericks HDB, Baldwin VL (1987) Individuals with sensory impairments. Who are they? How are they educated? In: Goetz L, Guess D, Stremel-Campbell K (eds) Innovative Program Design for Individuals with Dual Sensory Impairments. Brookes, Baltimore, MD, pp. 3–12.

Gee K, Harrell R, Rosenberg R (1987) Teaching orientation and mobility skills within and across natural opportunities for travel: a model designed for learners with multiple severe disabilities. In: Goetz L, Guess D, Stremel-Campbell K (eds) Innovative Program Design for Individuals with Dual Sensory Impairments. Brookes, Baltimore, MD, pp. 127–159.

Giangreco MF (2000) Related services research for students with low-incidence disabilities: Implications for speech-language pathologists in inclusive classrooms. Language, Speech and Hearing Service in Schools 31: 230–239.

Giangreco MF, Edelman SW, Nelson C (1998) Impact of planning for support services on students who are deaf-blind. Journal of Visual Impairment and Blindness 92: 18–29.

Giangreco MF, Edelman SW, Nelson C, Young MR, Kiefer-O Donnell R (1999) Changes in educational team membership for students who are deaf-blind in general education classes. Journal of Visual Impairment and Blindness 93: 166–173.

Godfrey NW, Costello MA (1995) Communication issues and strategies for deaf-blind individuals: case studies basic on etiology and language. American Rehabilitation 21: 40–45.

Goetz L, O'Farrell N (1999) Connections: facilitating social supports for students with deafblindness in general education classrooms. Journal of Visual Impairment and Blindness 93: 704–715.

Goode DA (1994) A World Without Words: The social construction of children born deaf and blind. Temple University Press, Philadelphia.

Greaves S (1999) Spiralling out in control. A model for service development for older people with acquired dual sensory impairment. Deafblind International Conference, 1999, Lisbon.

Gross ER (1994) Nonaversive olfactory conditioning to control aggressive behaviors of a blind, hearing impaired, and noncommunicating child. Journal of Developmental and Physical Disabilities 6: 77–82.

Hammer E (1978) Needs of adolescents who have Usher's syndrome. American Annals of the Deaf 123: 389–394.

Hammer E, Carlson R (1996) Using the intervener model with adults who are deaf-blind. Journal of Vocational Rehabilitation 7: 125–128.

Harrod MJE (1978) Genetic counselling for Usher's syndrome patients and their families. American Annals of the Deaf 123: 377–380.

Heller WK, Gallagher P-A, Fredrick L-D (1999) Parents' perceptions of siblings' interactions with their brothers and sisters who are deaf-blind. Journal of the Association for Persons with Severe Handicaps 24: 33–43.

Hess-Rover J, Crichton J, Byrne K, Holland AJ (1999) Diagnosis and treatment of a severe psychotic illness in a man with dual severe sensory impairments caused by the presence of Usher syndrome. Journal of Intellectual Disability Research 43: 428–434.

Hicks D (1978) Usher's syndrome: programmatic considerations. American Annals of the Deaf 123: 365–371.

Ingraham CL, Daugherty KM, Gorrafa S (1995) The success of three gifted deaf-blind students in inclusive educational programs. Journal of Visual Impairment and Blindness 89: 257–261.

Ingraham CL, Vernon M, Clemente B, Olney L (2000) Sex education for deaf-blind youths and adults. Journal of Visual Impairment and Blindness 94: 756–61.

Janssen MJ, Riksen-Walraven JM, Dijk JPM van (2002) Enhancing the quality of interaction between deafblind children and their educators. Journal of Developmental and Physical Disabilities 14: 87–109.

Janssen MJ, Riksen-Walraven JM, Dijk JPM van (2003) Contact: effects of an intervention program to foster harmonious interactions between deaf-blind children and their educators. Journal of Visual Impairment and Blindness 97: 215–229.

Kimberling WJ, Möller C (1995) Clinical and molecular genetics of Usher syndrome. Journal of the American Academy of Audiology 6: 63–72.

Kirchner C, Diament S (1999a) Estimates of the number of visually impaired students, their teachers, and orientation and mobility specialists: part 1. Journal of Visual Impairment and Blindness 93: 600–606.

Kirchner C, Diament S (1999b) Estimates of the number of visually impaired students, their teachers, and orientation and mobility specialists: part 2. Journal of Visual Impairment and Blindness 93: 738–744.

Lancioni GE, Mantini M (1999) A corrective-feedback system for helping a person with multiple disabilities during indoor travel. Perceptual and Motor Skills 88: 1291–1295.

Lancioni GE, Coninx F, Manders N, Driessen M (1991) Reducing breaks in performance of multihandicapped students through automatic prompting or peer supervision. Journal of Developmental and Physical Disabilities 3: 115–128.

Liberman LJ, Hugh BE (2001) Health related fitness of children who are visually impaired. Journal of Visual Impairment and Blindness 95: 272–287.

Liberman LJ, Stuart M (2002) Self-determined recreational and leisure choices of individual with deafblindness. Journal of Visual Impairment and Blindness 96: 724–735.

Liljedahl K (1993) Handikapp och omvärld – hundra års pedagogik för ett livslångt lärande [Handicap and environment – a hundred years of pedagogical efforts aimed at lifelong learning]. Department of Education, Lund University, Lund, Sweden.

Luiselli JK (1988) Positive reinforcement interventions in the classroom. Journal of Visual Impairment and Blindness 82: 17–20.

Luisclli JK (1991) A non-aversive behavioral pharmacological intervention for severe self-injury in an adult with dual sensory impairment. Journal of Behavior Therapy and Experimental Psychiatry 22: 233–238.

Luiselli JK (1992) Assessment and treatment of self-injury in a deaf-blind child. Journal of Developmental and Physical Disabilities 4: 219–226.

Luiselli JK, Lolli DA (1987) Contingency management of a blind child's disruptive behaviors during mobility instruction. Education of the Visually Handicapped 19: 65–70.

McDaniel G, Kocim R, Barton LE (1984) Reducing self-stimulatory mouthing behaviors in deaf-blind children. Journal of Visual Impairment and Blindness 78: 23–26.

MacFarland SZC (1995) Teaching strategies of the van Dijk curricular approach. Journal of Visual Impairment and Blindness 89: 222–228.

McInnes JM, Treffry JA (1982) Deaf-blind Infants and Children: A developmental guide. Open University Press, Buckingham, UK.

Mar HH, Sall N (1995) Enhancing social opportunities and relationships of children who are deaf-blind. Journal of Visual Impairment and Blindness 89: 280–286.

Marchant JM (1996) Deaf-blind. In: McLaughlin PJ, Wehman P (eds) Mental Retardation and Developmental Disabilities. Pro-Ed, Austin, TX.

Marks SB (1998) Understanding and preventing learned helplessness in children who are congenitally deaf-blind. Journal of Visual Impairment and Blindness 92: 200–211.

Mesch J (1998) Teckenspråk i taktil form Turtagning och frågor i dövblindas samtal på teckenspråk (in Swedish). Institutionen för lingvistik Stockholms Universitet, Stockholm, Sweden.

Miner I (1999) Psychotherapy for people with Usher syndrome. In: Leigh IW (ed.) Psychotherapy with Deaf Clients from Diverse Groups. Gallaudet University Press, Washington, DC, pp. 307–327.

Miner ID (1995) Psychosocial implications of Usher syndrome, type I, throughout the life cycle. Journal of Visual Impairment and Blindness 89: 287–296.

Miner ID (1996) The impact of Usher's syndrome, type I on adolescent development. Journal of Vocational Rehabilitation 6: 159–166.

Miner ID (1997) People with Usher syndrome, type II: issues and adaptations. Journal of Visual Impairment and Blindness 91: 579–589.

Miner ID, Feldman MD (1998) Factitious deafblindness: an imperceptible variant of factitious disorder. General Hospital Psychiatry 20: 48–51.

Murdoch H (1994) The development of infants who are deaf-blind: a case study. Journal of Visual Impairment and Blindness 88: 357–367.

Myrbakk E (1991) The treatment of self-stimulation of a severely mentally retarded and deaf-blind client by brief physical interruption: a case report. Scandinavian Journal of Behaviour Therapy 20: 41.

Nafstad AV, Rödbroe IB (1999) Co-creating Communication. Forlaget-Nord Press, Oslo.

Parsons MB, Reid DH, Green CW (1998) Identifying work preferences prior to supported work for an individual with multiple severe disabilities including deafblindness. Journal of the Association for Persons with Severe Handicaps 23: 329–333.

Peine HA, Liu L, Blakelock H, Jenson WR, Osborne JG (1991) The use of contingent water misting in the treatment of self-choking. Journal of Behavior Therapy and Experimental Psychiatry 22: 225-231.

Petroff JG (2001) National Transition Follow-Up Study Of Youth Identified As Deafblind: Parents' Perspective. Retrieved 13 May 2003 from www.tr.wou.edu/ntac/transition. htm.

Petronio K (1988) Interpreting for deaf-blind students: factors to consider. American Annals of the Deaf 133: 226-229.

Pollard RQ, Miner ID, Cioffi J (2000) Hearing and vision loss. In: Frank RG, Timothy TR (eds) Handbook of Rehabilitation Psychology. American Psychological Association, Washington, DC, pp. 205-234.

Rapoff MA, Altman K, Christopherson-Edward R (1980) Suppression of self-injurious behaviour: determining the least restrictive alternative. Journal of Mental Deficiency Research 24: 37-46.

Reed CM, Rabinowitz WM, Durlach NI et al. (1985) Research on the Tadoma method of speech communication. Journal of the Acoustical Society of America 77: 247-257.

Reed CM, Delhorne LA, Durlach NI, Fischer SD (1990) A study of the tactual and visual reception of fingerspelling. Journal of Speech and Hearing Research 33: 786-797.

Reed CM, Delhorne LA, Durlach NI, Fischer SD (1995) A study of the tactual reception of sign language. Journal of Speech and Hearing Research 38: 477-489.

Reed HL, Fontan LE (1987) A model program to determine the needs of deaf-blind persons. Journal of Rehabilitation of the Deaf 21: 16-17.

Romer LT, Schoenberg B (1991) Increasing requests made by people with developmental disabilities and deafblindness through the use of behavior interruption strategies. Education and Training in Mental Retardation 26: 70-78.

Rönnberg J, Borg E (2001) A review and evaluation of research on the deaf-blind from perceptual, communicative, social, and rehabilitative perspectives. Scandinavian Audiology 30: 67-77.

Rönnberg J, Samuelsson E, Borg E (2002) Exploring the perceived world of the deaf-blind: on the development of an instrument. International Journal of Audiology 41: 136-143.

Sauerburger D, Jones S (1997) Corner to corner: how can deaf-blind travellers solicit aid effectively? Rehabilitation and Education for Blindness and Visual Impairment 29: 34-44.

Siegel-Causey E, Downing J (1987) Nonsymbolic communication development. In: Goetz L, Guess D, Stremel-Campbell K (eds) Innovative Program Design for Individuals with Dual Sensory Impairments. Brookes, Baltimore, MD, pp. 15-48.

Sisson LA, Hersen M, Van-Hasselt VB (1993) Improving the performance of youth with dual sensory impairment: Analyses and social validation of procedures to reduce maladaptive responding in vocational and leisure settings. Behavior Therapy 24: 553-571.

Statens sentralteam (1999) Rapport fra prosjektet Kartlegging av eldre mennesker med allvorlig kombinert syns- og hörselnedsettelse oppföging veiledning informasjon (in Norwegian). Statens sentralteam for døvblinde, Oslo.

Stein LK, Palmer P, Weinberg B (1982) Characteristics of a young deaf-blind population. American Annals of the Deaf 127: 828-837.

Stoop JA (1996) Deafblindness in the elderly leading to psycho-social problems. Nederlands Tijdschrift voor Geneeskunde 140: 1845-1848.

Tedder NE (1987) Counselling issues for clients with Usher's syndrome. Journal of Rehabilitation 53: 61-64.

Torrie C (1978) Families of adolescent children with Usher's syndrome: developing service to meet their needs. American Annals of the Deaf 123: 381-388.

Tweedie D (1974) Demonstrating behavioral change of deaf-blind children. Exceptional Children 40: 510-512.

Vernon M (1969) Usher's syndrome: deafness and progressive blindness – clinical cases, prevention, theory and literature survey. Journal of Chronic Disease 22: 133-151.

Vernon M, Duncan E (1990) Advances in rehabilitation of deaf-blind persons. Advances in Clinical Rehabilitation 3: 167-184.

Vernon M, Hammer E (1996) The state of the evaluation and diagnosis of deaf-blind people: psychological and functional approaches. Journal of Vocational Rehabilitation 6: 133-141.

Watkins S, Clark T, Strong C, Barringer D (1994) The effectiveness of an intervener model of services for young deaf-blind children. American Annals of the Deaf 139: 404-409.

Wolf-Schein EG (1989) A review of the size, characteristics, and needs of the deaf-blind population of North America. ACEHI Journal 15: 85-89.

Yarnall GD (1980) Teaching a deaf-blind woman to 'wait' on command. Journal of Visual Impairment and Blindness 74: 24-27.

Yarnall GD, Dodgion-Ensor B (1980) Identifying effective reinforcers for a multiply handicapped student. Education of the Visually Handicapped 12: 11-20.

CHAPTER 9
The effects of otosclerosis

NELE LEMKENS

Otosclerosis is a very frequent cause of hearing loss. Abnormal bone homoeostasis causes lesions in the otic capsule. These foci of otosclerotic bone have no functional consequence until the stapedial movements are impaired by invasion of the stapedovestibular joint, causing a conductive hearing loss. It is believed that in the later stages of the disease, otosclerosis also affects the inner ear causing additional sensorineural hearing loss (Schuknecht and Kirchner, 1974; Kelemen and Alonso, 1980).

In the large group of genetically determined hearing losses, otosclerosis is a unique disease because it is primarily conductive in nature. People tend to perceive a conductive hearing loss differently from a sensorineural hearing loss, because, among other reasons, the former is eligible for surgery. The fact that it is 'remediable' also makes it less popular as a subject in literature about psychosocial consequences of hearing loss. The literature on otosclerosis surgery, on the other hand, is enormous. However, surgeons rarely use patient satisfaction instruments to measure the outcome of their surgery. Little interest from both groups – psychological and social science professionals as well as otological surgeons – has created a gap in our knowledge about the psychosocial consequences of otosclerosis.

The genetic nature of otosclerosis is complicated and only partly known at present. The prevalence of clinical otosclerosis in the white population can be estimated as 3/1000 (Declau et al., 2001). Investigation of the pedigrees of families with otosclerosis has shown that it is an autosomal dominant disease with a reduced penetrance of 40%. To date, three different otosclerosis-causing genes have been localized in otosclerosis families, although no causative genes have yet been cloned. Still, in 30–50% of all patients with clinical otosclerosis there is no family history of hearing loss (Gordon, 1989). It is difficult to explain the existence of so many sporadic cases on the basis of reduced penetrance alone. An autosomal recessive mode of inheritance has been proposed for these cases, but nowadays otosclerosis is more and more considered as a complex disease, where there is an interaction between several genes and different environmental triggers (Van Den Bogaert et al., 2002). Monogenic otosclerosis families would then be the exception rather than the rule.

The impact of otosclerosis on the basis of the ICF framework

The aim of this chapter is to give an overview of the existing literature on the psychosocial consequences of otosclerosis, following the ICF framework (WHO, 2001). As already mentioned, literature on this subject is scarce, so some information was drawn from publications about conductive hearing loss in general. Publications on otosclerosis surgery using patient satisfaction instruments also yielded some indirect information.

Hearing and related functions; activity limitations

Patients with otosclerosis mainly suffer from conductive hearing loss. Because frequency and temporal resolution are generally unaltered, otosclerotic patients have less difficulty understanding speech in noise as compared to patients with a sensorineural hearing loss of equivalent degree. However, theoretically, the recruitment typically seen in sensorineural hearing loss could have a relevant advantage at moderate intensities. Gatehouse and Haggard (1987) showed that, for word identification at low stimulus levels, the patient with conductive hearing loss suffers a greater disability for a given hearing loss. At high levels they report less disability. The crossover point between these regions (i.e. where a single predictor from hearing level correctly predicts equal disability for those with conductive and sensorineural hearing loss) is approximately 85 dB SPL (sound pressure level). Lutman, Brown and Coles (1987) have reported that scaled responses on a disability questionnaire show relatively greater disability in conductive than sensorineural loss, once respondents' air conduction threshold levels are taken into account. Ayache, Earally and Elbaz (2003) found that in 75% of patients with otosclerosis there is a low-pitched tinnitus. A questionnaire revealed that 25% of the patients find the tinnitus severely disabling. Eriksson-Mangold, Erlandsson and Jansson (1996) reported on tinnitus in patients with otosclerosis, on the basis of focus-group interviews. Here also tinnitus appeared to be a major problem for some patients; some of them even regarded the tinnitus as more of a problem than the hearing loss itself.

Participation restriction

Two groups of researchers have investigated otosclerosis from a psychological point of view. Gildston and Gildston (1972) used a 'temperament survey' to profile the personality of 37 patients with otosclerosis. The survey was administered pre- and postoperatively. Preoperatively, subjects' scores were significantly impaired for the traits of friendliness, ascendancy, sociability, emotional stability, objectivity, personal relations and also masculinity for the males. Scores for all traits except masculinity were significantly better postoperatively. Also, mean scores on an 'optimism–pessimism scale' measured postoperatively were significantly better than the mean score measured preoperatively.

Jasovic Gasic et al. (1991) administered two different surveys to 40 patients with otosclerosis and 16 control subjects. They also found psychopathological disturbances in 30% of the patients, compared with 18.7% of the control subjects.

Stewart (2001) developed a disease-specific hearing status instrument for use in conductive hearing loss: the Hearing Satisfaction Scale (HSS). A short questionnaire has to be completed by the subject. The total score can be divided into an emotional subscore and a social/situational subscore. In this study 89 patients with conductive hearing losses (including 73 people with otosclerosis) were evaluated with this instrument and with the SF-36 (a general quality-of-life measure), before any intervention and after an operation or fitting with a hearing aid. The SF-36 was not sensitive to changes in hearing loss, but the HSS was. Intervention (mostly surgery) improved scores on the HSS significantly, but did not bring them to a level comparable to healthy adults. It did result in the HSS correlating better with the SF-36.

Personal contextual factors

Some personal factors that could influence the individual's degree of activity limitation and participation restriction are quoted by Stewart (2001). People with a conductive hearing loss are mostly younger than those with a sensorineural hearing loss. This also holds true for otosclerotic patients, where the age of onset generally lies between 15 and 45 years of age. Because of their age these patients typically do not have other sensory (e.g. loss of vision) or cognitive deficits. In general they are more active in their professional and social lives.

Attitudes towards surgery and its impact

Eriksson-Mangold, Erlandsson and Jansson (1996) conducted focus-group interviews to estimate the subjective meaning of illness in severe otosclerosis. They tried to identify aspects of the disease, other than the functional hearing loss, that have an impact on psychosocial functioning. Surgery appeared to be central to the concerns of patients with otosclerosis. The fact that their disease is 'curable' implies that they have to take responsibility because they have to decide for or against surgery. This feeling of being able to act on the disease can make it easier to adapt to the disease, but it can also be a great burden to have to make the decision for or against surgery. An operation also means that the patient can get his hearing back. This is a very happy event, but it also causes the patient to worry that it might 'break' again. The possibility of surgery makes the disease more understandable for others and gives rise to feelings of sympathy. After surgery the patient has to adjust to the new sound level (it cannot be turned off). At the very beginning most people feel that all the new sounds are tiring and irritating. Finally, because of the possibility of an operation, hearing aids are regarded as 'second best'.

In the literature about otosclerosis surgery, the main outcome measures are air–bone gap closure and pure-tone threshold improvement. Reported postoperative results from these studies are invariably excellent. However, these measures do not necessarily assess whether the patient has benefited. Fortunately there seems to be a trend to take the hearing in the non-operated ear into account when reporting postoperative results (e.g. the Glasgow Benefit Plot). This has encouraged surgeons to look at the results of their surgery from a more functional standpoint, rather than in purely technical terms. Many other factors such as sound distortion and hyperacusis or dizziness influence patient satisfaction and quality of life after surgery. A few publications about stapes surgery have used patient satisfaction as an outcome measure.

A more in-depth analysis of factors influencing patient satisfaction after surgery was conducted by Ramsay, Karkkainen and Palva (1997). They retrospectively investigated the results of 270 stapes operations, looking at audiometric results. They also asked patients for their evaluation of hearing and benefits of surgery, and questioned them about subjective symptoms such as tinnitus, vertigo, loudness intolerance, pain, chorda tympani symptoms and sound distortion problems. Subjectively, 79.5% of the patients rated their hearing improvement as 'considerable'. Subjective evaluation of benefit correlated significantly with the objective audiometric results: 52% had postoperative tinnitus, 19.6% had vertigo, 18.5% had occasional pain in the operated ear, 35.2% had loud noise intolerance, 26.3% had occasional sound distortion, 14.4% had postoperative chorda tympani symptoms, mostly transient. Subjective symptoms and complaints significantly affected the patients' opinion of the general benefit from surgery, although a considerable hearing improvement appeared to compensate for most postoperative subjective complaints.

Lundman et al. (1999) conducted a similar investigation. They studied 95 patients undergoing unilateral surgery for otosclerosis and studied the self-assessment of hearing and audiometric results. Interestingly, they asked patients to recall how disabled they were preoperatively because of their hearing. This question, although imperfect, can teach us something about the influence of the hearing impairment caused by otosclerosis itself, without any contamination by surgical procedures. It appeared that most patients experienced profound social hearing disability regardless of whether they had unilateral or bilateral hearing loss. At home, however, patients with bilateral hearing loss were much more likely to experience severe hearing disability than did those with a unilateral hearing loss. A hearing loss greater than 40 dB in one ear, even with the other ear normal, appeared to be a strong predictor for hearing problems in social situations. Despite acceptable surgical results in 95% of patients, only 64% had satisfactory social hearing at follow-up. In this study patients only had unilateral surgery. The authors concluded that the other ear, left with poor hearing, was responsible for the difference between objective and subjective results. This would indicate that plots taking into account the hearing in both ears are indeed useful in predicting outcome of otosclerosis surgery.

Family

No investigations of the influence of having a positive family history of otosclerosis on the psychosocial consequences of the condition have been conducted. As part of a genetic programme we investigated a family with several cases of severe otosclerosis, some of whom had received a cochlear implant in the end-stage of their disease. Nine affected subjects completed a questionnaire about psychosocial consequences of their hearing loss. One question asked *how* they were influenced by the fact that other family members had the same kind of hearing problem. All but one answered that this had influenced them in a positive way. A further open-ended question asked *why* they were influenced by the fact that they had other family members with the same problem. They answered that it had helped them to be prepared, even in a practical way – planning their work, for example. They also found that the problem could easily be discussed in the family, and that the problem of hearing loss could not be understood by somebody with normal hearing. A negative consequence was that they were very afraid their children would also be affected.

Conclusions

Otosclerosis is a very common disease and is familial in 50% of cases. The fact that the hearing loss is mostly conductive in nature makes it unique in the large group of genetic hearing impairments. A conductive hearing loss has other audiological features: for instance, there is no recruitment and no distortion of temporal or frequency resolution. Afflicted people are younger and more active in their professional and social lives. However, the possibility of surgery seems to be the most important feature distinguishing otosclerosis from sensorineural hearing loss. Operations are central to the concerns of patients with otosclerosis. Surgeons should take into account the hearing in both ears in order to achieve better functional outcome. Other symptoms such as sound distortion and tinnitus are also important for the patients' subjective opinion of the surgical outcome. However, only a limited amount of information is available and much more research is needed. Health workers other than surgeons should investigate the patients' attitudes to otosclerosis. The influence of having a family history of the condition has not been thoroughly investigated, but it appears that this helps the patients to cope with their hearing loss.

References

Ayache D, Earally F, Elbaz P (2003) Characteristics and postoperative course of tinnitus in otosclerosis. Otology and Neurotology 24: 48–51.

Declau F, Spaendonck M Van, Timmermans JP et al. (2001) Prevalence of otosclerosis in an unselected series of temporal bones. Otology and Neurotology 22: 596–602.

Eriksson-Mangold M, Erlandsson SI, Jansson G (1996) The subjective meaning of illness in severe otosclerosis: a descriptive study in three steps based on focus group interviews and written questionnaire. Scandinavian Audiology, Supplementum 43: 34–44.

Gatehouse S, Haggard MP (1987) The effects of air-bone gap and presentation level on word identification. Ear and Hearing 8: 140–146.

Gildston H, Gildston P (1972) Personality changes associated with surgically corrected hypoacusis. Audiology 11: 354–367.

Gordon MA (1989) The genetics of otosclerosis: a review. American Journal of Otology 10: 426–438.

Jasovic Gasic M, Leposavic L, Savic D et al. (1991) Psychological aspects of hearing loss in otosclerosis. Psychiatria Danubina 3: 495–511.

Kelemen G, Alonso A (1980) Penetration of the cochlear endost by the fibrous component of the otosclerotic focus. Acta Otolaryngologica 89: 453–458.

Lundman L, Mendel L, Bagger-Sjoback D, Rosenhall U (1999) Hearing in patients operated unilaterally for otosclerosis. Self-assessment of hearing and audiometric results. Acta Otolaryngologica 119: 453–458.

Lutman ME, Brown EJ, Coles RR (1987) Self-reported disability and handicap in the population in relation to pure-tone threshold, age, sex and type of hearing loss. British Journal of Audiology 21: 45–58.

Ramsay H, Karkkainen J, Palva T (1997) Success in surgery for otosclerosis: hearing improvement and other indicators. American Journal of Otology 18: 23–28.

Schuknecht HF, Kirchner JC (1974) Cochlear otosclerosis: fact or fantasy. Laryngoscope 84: 766–782.

Stewart MG (2001) Outcomes and patient-based hearing status in conductive hearing loss. Laryngoscope 111: 1–21.

Van Den Bogaert K, Govaerts PJ, Leenheer EM De et al. (2002) Otosclerosis: a genetically heterogeneous disease involving at least three different genes. Bone 30: 624–630.

WHO (2001) International Classification of Functioning, Disability and Health – ICF. World Health Organization, Geneva, Switzerland.

CHAPTER 10
Psychosocial aspects of neurofibromatosis type 2

WANDA NEARY, RICHARD RAMSDEN, GARETH EVANS AND
MICHAEL BASER

Neurofibromatosis type 2 (NF2) is a dominantly inherited genetic condition caused by a defect on chromosome 22. Approximately 50% of cases have a family history of NF2 and show clearly dominant transmission. In the remaining cases the condition arises as a result of a new mutation. The hallmark of NF2 is the presence of bilateral vestibular Schwannomas, but meningiomas, gliomas and ependymomas are associated with the disorder. Schwannomas may occur in the spinal canal and on peripheral nerves. Total deafness is likely in most cases as a result of tumours of the eighth cranial nerve, or surgery to remove them. Premature death is common in the most severely affected individuals, but in some patients the progression of the condition is slow and the patients retain hearing into their seventies. There is a high probability of lens abnormalities in individuals with NF2, and slit-lamp examination of the lenses through dilated pupils may reveal presenile lenticular opacities and cortical opacities. Cutaneous examination may reveal the presence of café-au-lait macules, but nearly always fewer than six in number. The incidence of tumours of the central and peripheral nervous systems, together with the cutaneous and ophthalmological findings from three large studies of patients with NF2 (Evans et al., 1992a; Parry et al., 1994; Mautner et al., 1996), is documented in Table 10.1.

Individuals affected with NF2 may be expected to experience an impact on their lives due to the disorder, particularly in the areas designated as *participation* and *personal factors* as defined in the International Classification of Functioning, Disability and Health [ICF]; see Chapter 3). In NF2 there are four major areas to be considered: hearing impairment, disfigurement, mobility and vision. There are effects of progressive hearing impairment on the individual, together with the possibility of postoperative cosmetic sequelae from facial palsy. Peripheral neuropathy is a well-recognized feature of NF2 in adults, but mononeuropathy is a condition that

Table 10.1. The age at onset, frequency of tumour types, and cutaneous and ocular features in NF2

	Evans et al. (1992a)	Parry et al. (1994)	Mautner et al. (1996)
Number of cases	120	63	48
Number of families	75	32	Not stated
Isolated cases	45	17	44
Age at onset (years)	22.2	20.3	17
Meningiomas	45%	49%	58%
Spinal tumours	25.8%	67%	90%
Skin tumours	68% (of 100 cases)	67%	64%
More than 10 skin tumours	10% (of 100 cases)	Not known	Not known
Café-au-lait macules	43% (of 100 cases)	47%	42%
Cataracts	38% (of 90 cases)	81%	62%
Astrocytoma	4.1%	1.6%	15%
Ependymoma	2.5%	3.2%	6%
Optic sheath meningioma	4.1%	4.8%	8%

occurs primarily in children (Evans, Birch and Ramsden, 1999). There is a high incidence of amblyopia in NF2, together with presenile cataracts. Early third nerve neuropathy, and fifth and seventh nerve damage may occur. A further area to consider is whether the individual has received an auditory brain-stem implant (ABI), and whether they feel that they have benefited from the device. The effects of genetic counselling and support organizations should be taken into account. The impact of the diagnosis of NF2 on the partner and family should be given careful consideration.

Historical background

In 1822 the Scottish surgeon Wishart described a patient with subcutaneous tumours, bilateral deafness, blindness, headache and vomiting. At autopsy the patient was found to have tumours in the skull, dura mater and brain. Wishart's publication was probably the first documented account of a patient with NF2. The classic description of neurofibromatosis was made by the German pathologist von Recklinghausen in 1882. He described two of his own patients who had multiple skin and subcutaneous tumours, and who also exhibited numerous large pigmented skin patches. He reviewed three further cases from the literature. The term 'neurofibromatosis' was introduced by von Recklinghausen as he recognized that neural elements were present in both cutaneous and subcutaneous tumours. He emphasized that one patient had an affected relative, and realized that the condition was familial rather than acquired.

Henschen (1910, 1915) suggested that bilateral vestibular tumours were associated with von Recklinghausen's disease. Between 1910 and 1915 he described a total of 245 cases of unilateral vestibular tumours and 24 cases of bilateral vestibular tumours. Mild skin changes of von Recklinghausen's disease were found in 19 out of the 24 cases with bilateral vestibular tumours but in only 5 out of the 245 cases with unilateral vestibular tumours. The association of bilateral vestibular tumours and von Recklinghausen's disease was supported by Cushing in 1917 and Fraser in 1921.

In 1930 Gardner and Frazier published a clinical study and field survey of a family of 5 generations with bilateral deafness in 38 members. They suggested that bilateral vestibular tumours represented a separate central form of von Recklinghausen's disease.

In 1940 Gardner and Turner published a further report on the same family. One of the affected individuals had developed a tumour of the spinal cord, which proved to be a neurofibroma. Meningiomas were observed to occur in association with bilateral vestibular tumours. They observed that there was minimal evidence of peripheral neurofibromatosis.

Young, Eldridge and Gardner (1970) found that peripheral signs suggestive of neurofibromatosis were rare in patients with bilateral vestibular tumours, but other central nervous system tumours, often asymptomatic, were common.

In 1980 Kanter et al. published a genetic, clinical and biochemical study of nine families in which two or more individuals had the central form of neurofibromatosis. They stated that their findings suggested that neurofibromatosis was a syndrome consisting of at least two forms, peripheral and central. They suggested that the term 'von Recklinghausen's disease' should be reserved for the peripheral form, since the German pathologist did not describe cases of central neurofibromatosis.

A clear distinction between NF1 and NF2 was not made until 1987. By that year genetic linkage studies had resulted in the mapping of the gene for NF1 to chromosome 17 (Barker et al., 1987), and the gene for NF2 to chromosome 22 (Rouleau et al., 1987; Seizinger et al., 1987a). The National Institutes of Health (NIH) Consensus Development Conference on Neurofibromatosis held in 1987 discussed the question of nomenclature and classification, and concluded that there was sufficient evidence to clearly distinguish two forms of neurofibromatosis, NF1 and NF2. The NIH Consensus statement published in 1988 formally separated the two conditions.

Bilateral vestibular tumours were said to occur in 2–4% of individuals with von Recklinghausen's neurofibromatosis (Crowe, Schull and Neel, 1956). Huson, Compston and Harper (1989) carried out a population-based study of NF1 using the internationally agreed diagnostic criteria (National Institutes of Health, 1987) to determine whether vestibular Schwannomas occurred in NF1. No cases of vestibular Schwannomas were found in 135 individuals with NF1.

Diagnostic criteria

Diagnostic criteria for NF2 were agreed by the NIH Consensus Development Conference on Neurofibromatosis in 1987. Additional criteria were described by Evans et al. (1992a) to allow for individuals with multiple intracranial and spinal tumours, but not bilateral vestibular Schwannomas (Evans et al., 1992b). The NIH criteria, and those of Evans and co-workers, are presented in Table 10.2.

Table 10.2. Diagnostic criteria for NF2

NIH criteria (1987)
A diagnosis of NF2 is made in a patient who has:
* Bilateral vestibular Schwannomas
* Or a family history of NF2
* Plus a unilateral vestibular Schwannoma
* Or any two of: meningioma, glioma, neurofibroma, Schwannoma, posterior subcapsular lenticular opacities

Additional criteria (Evans et al., 1992b)
A diagnosis of NF2 can also be made in a patient who has:
* A unilateral vestibular Schwannoma
* Plus any two of: meningioma, glioma, neurofibroma, Schwannoma, posterior subcapsular lenticular opacities
* Or multiple meningiomas (two or more)
* Plus a unilateral vestibular Schwannoma
* Or any two of: glioma, neurofibroma, Schwannoma, cataract

Baser et al. (2002a) evaluated four previous sets of clinical diagnostic criteria for NF2 developed by international groups of experts: the NIH criteria (1987); the Consensus Development Panel of the NIH (1991); the Manchester Group criteria reported by Evans et al. (1992b); and the National Neurofibromatosis Foundation (NNFF) 1997 criteria, reported by Gutmann et al. (1997). Baser and co-workers reported that none of the existing sets of criteria was adequate at initial assessment for diagnosing individuals who presented without bilateral vestibular Schwannomas, particularly individuals without a family history of NF2.

Epidemiology

NF2 has a birth incidence of 1 in 35 000–40 000 in the UK (Evans et al., 1992c). However, the actual diagnostic prevalence is only 1 in 210 000 as many individuals do not develop features of the condition until the third decade or later, and other individuals with aggressive disease die before the third decade. An annual incidence rate of 1 per 2355 000 was reported by Evans et al. (1993).

Presenting symptoms

Most adults with NF2 present with hearing loss, tinnitus, and imbalance and vertigo, related to the presence of bilateral vestibular Schwannomas. Kanter et al. (1980) described bilateral hearing loss as the most common initial symptom, reported in half of their 124 cases. Subsequent studies by Martuza and Eldridge (1988), Evans et al. (1992a), Neary et al. (1993) and Parry et al. (1994) described unilateral hearing loss as the first symptom to be noted in individuals with NF2.

Evans et al. (1992a) reported on 150 patients with NF2. The average age of onset of symptoms in 110 cases was 21.6 years and at diagnosis 27.5 years. Mean age at death in 40 cases was 36.2 years, but including the living cases mean actuarial survival was 62 years. Mean actuarial survival from diagnosis was 15 years. In the north-west of England, where there were 19 living cases, mean age at onset was 26.5 years and at diagnosis 30.5 years, showing that ascertainment bias was not causing identification of only severely affected cases from the remainder of the UK. In 100 patients, Evans et al. reported that 44 presented with hearing impairment, which was unilateral in 35 and was accompanied by tinnitus in 10. Muscle weakness or wasting was the first symptom in 12%. A distal symmetrical sensorimotor neuropathy, confirmed by nerve conduction studies and electromyography, was found in 3 out of the 100 patients. The authors reported that, although similar features could result from the multiple spinal and intracranial tumours in NF2, a generalized or isolated neuropathy appeared to be a relatively common feature. They found 34 out of 90 patients to have cataracts, 4 probably being congenital.

Evans et al. (1992a) described two types of patients with NF2, the Wishart type and the Gardner type. The Wishart type presented at an early age, the disease progression was rapid, and the patient had multiple other tumours in addition to bilateral vestibular Schwannomas. In contrast, the Gardner type occurred at a later age, had a more benign course, and usually only bilateral vestibular Schwannomas.

Parry et al. (1994) evaluated 63 individuals affected with NF2 from 32 families. The mean age at onset in 58 individuals was 20.3 years. In 44.4% initial symptoms were related to vestibular Schwannoms; in 22.2% the first symptoms were related to other tumours of the central nervous system. Cataracts affected 81% of individuals, skin tumours were present in 67.7%, spinal tumours in 67.4% and meningiomas in 49.2%. Parry et al. noted that clinical manifestations and the clinical course were similar within families, but differed between families.

Mautner et al. (1996) performed gadolinium-enhanced magnetic resonance imaging (MRI) of the brain and spine as well as neurological, dermatological and ocular examinations in 48 patients with NF2 diagnosed by the NIH diagnostic criteria. The presenting symptoms included hearing loss or tinnitus in 31% of patients, multiple or non-specific symptoms in 31%, skin tumours in 25% and ocular symptoms in 13%. The mean age at onset of symptoms was 17 years. Vestibular Schwannomas were found in 96% of patients and meningiomas in 58%. Mautner et al. commented that it was noteworthy that, when the complete spine was imaged, spinal tumours were more common in patients with NF2 than had previously been reported.

MacCollin and Mautner (1998) drew attention to the fact that the presentation and natural history of NF2 differ in children and adults, with eighth nerve dysfunction in children often overshadowed by the effects of other tumours on the nervous system. These authors stated that most adults present with symptoms referable to vestibular Schwannomas, and auditory symptoms predominate over vestibular. In contrast, they found that children were much more likely to present with other neurological symptoms, primarily those of spinal cord compression or visual dysfunction.

Evans, Birch and Ramsden (1999) reported that the pattern of presentation in children aged 10 years or younger was very different from that of adults presenting with NF2. Hearing loss and tinnitus were the presenting symptoms in 20% of children in their series. However, children frequently presented with symptoms of an isolated tumour: 19 out of 61 children presented with symptoms of a meningioma – 7 with a spinal tumour and 5 with a cutaneous tumour. The authors drew attention to the fact that 6 children presented with a unilateral facial palsy. This high percentage of facial palsy at presentation in childhood contrasts with a facial weakness at presentation of 2% or less in a series of more than 650 histologically confirmed vestibular Schwannomas in adult patients (Ramsden, 1999, unpublished data). As mononeuropathies and a more widespread peripheral neuropathy are recognized features of NF2, Evans et al. suggested that this might be the cause of at least some of the facial palsies in childhood NF2. The authors also reported that two of their children presented with a foot drop. In one case a normal result was obtained on a spinal MRI scan, excluding a spinal tumour as a cause of the foot drop.

Baser et al. (2002b) analysed the mortality experience of 368 patients from 261 families in the UK NF2 registry, to evaluate clinical predictors of the risk of mortality in individuals with NF2. The age at diagnosis, intracranial meningiomas and type of treatment centre were predictors of the risk of mortality. The relative risk of mortality increased 1.13-fold for each year of decrease in age at diagnosis, and was 2.51-fold greater in people with meningiomas compared with those without meningiomas. The relative risk of mortality in patients treated at specialist centres was 0.34, compared with those treated at non-specialist centres.

Diagnosis

NF2 can be diagnosed if the criteria in Table 10.2 are satisfied. However, there are individuals who should be considered to be at risk of NF2, and should be investigated. High-risk individuals include those with a family history of NF2, those presenting with a unilateral vestibular Schwannoma or meningioma when aged 30 years or younger, patients with multiple spinal Schwannomas and meningiomas, and individuals with minimal skin features of neurofibromatosis insufficient for a diagnosis of NF1.

MRI with gadolinium enhancement provides the gold standard in diagnostic terms, with the possibility of revealing tumours as small as 2–3 mm in size (Welling and Glasscock, 1992). A cranial scan should be undertaken, together with a complete spinal scan.

Presymptomatic DNA diagnosis of NF2 can be undertaken using molecular genetic techniques.

Genetics

Seizinger, Martuza and Gusella (1986) demonstrated that specific loss of genes on chromosome 22 was a frequent occurrence in cases of sporadic vestibular Schwannomas. Tumours from patients with bilateral vestibular Schwannomas were investigated, and specific loss of constitutional heterozygosity for chromosome 22 was found in the hereditary condition. It was further demonstrated that in these patients specific loss of alleles from chromosome 22 occurred in two neurofibromas and one meningioma. This suggested a common pathogenic mechanism for the three tumour types (Seizinger et al., 1987b). Further studies of both sporadically occurring tumours and tumours from NF2 patients provided consistent support for the hypothesis that the NF2 locus encoded a recessive tumour-suppressor gene, where inactivation of both copies of the gene led to tumour formation (Rouleau et al., 1990).

Linkage studies assigned the NF2 gene to chromosome 22 (Rouleau et al., 1987; Wertelecki et al., 1988; Rouleau et al., 1990; Narod et al., 1992). The combined use of family studies and tumour deletion mapping progressively narrowed the location of the NF2 gene within the q12 band of chromosome 22 (Rouleau et al., 1990; Wolff et al., 1992).

A candidate gene for the NF2 tumour suppressor that had suffered non-overlapping deletions in DNA in four independent NF2 patients was identified. This candidate gene encoded a novel protein related to the moesin–ezrin–radixin family of cytoskeleton-associated proteins (Sato et al., 1992) and was named merlin (Trofatter et al., 1993) or schwannomin (Rouleau et al., 1993).

Molecular genetic techniques such as single-strand conformation polymorphism (SSCP) analysis or denaturing gradient gel electrophoresis (DGGE) detect 35–60% of causative mutations (Bourn et al., 1994; MacCollin et al., 1994; Merel et al., 1995). Zucman-Rossi et al. (1998) described a mutation screening strategy which has raised the efficiency of mutation detection in NF2 patients to 84% of the cases in their series.

There have been several reports on genotype–phenotype correlations with truncating mutations, where a partial gene product may be produced, and a more severe phenotype has been found. In contrast, a mild phenotype is seen in most missense mutations, which give rise to a complete protein product, or deletions, which give no protein product.

Parry et al. (1996) identified mutations in the NF2 gene in 66% of 32 patients. In 21 patients 20 different mutations were identified. They reported that, in patients with clinical manifestations compatible with severe disease, molecular genetic analysis had identified nonsense and frameshift mutations.

Ruttledge et al. (1996) reported that 24 out of 28 patients with mutations that cause premature truncation of the NF2 protein presented with clinical manifestations of severe NF2. This was in contrast to all 16 cases from 3 families who had mild disease, where the mutations were found to affect only a single amino acid.

In the vast majority of families where there are two or more living individuals who are affected with NF2, predictive diagnosis is possible by linkage analysis using flanking markers (Narod et al., 1992; Ruttledge et al., 1993; Evans et al., 1995). Linkage analysis will give greater than 99% certainty by using intragenic or flanking markers.

Standard mutation detection techniques (SSCP or DGGE) may detect the causative mutation in an individual affected with NF2. In such an instance a 100% specific test is available for the family. The disadvantage of this approach is that mutation detection is time-consuming and expensive, and the causative mutation is not identified in every individual affected with NF2.

Management and treatment

Individuals with NF2 present many complex considerations in diagnosis, medical and surgical management, and genetic counselling. Evans et al. (1993) emphasized the importance of multidisciplinary regional or supraregional centres with experience in dealing with all aspects of NF2, with input from neuro-otologists, neurosurgeons, ophthalmologists, geneticists, audiologists, speech therapists, counsellors, psychologists and occasionally psychiatrists being recommended.

Bance and Ramsden (1999) advised that the treatment plan must include screening of relatives and genetic counselling. Before 1993 only a minority of NF2 patients received genetic counselling (Evans et al., 1992b). Bance and Ramsden emphasized that the physician should be sensitive to the psychological impact of NF2 as a potentially devastating disease for the affected individual and the family. They stated that the impact is particularly marked in those families in which the disorder appears for the first time as a new mutation, and parental anxieties and guilt feelings are common. Bance and Ramsden stated that the physician must ensure, as much as possible, that the patient is prepared for the psychological blow of eventual total hearing loss and initiate appropriate training in non-auditory communication skills when necessary. They suggested that the challenge in the management of individuals affected with NF2 is to arrive at a treatment strategy that preserves useful hearing and quality of life without increasing the risk of complications to the facial nerve, or compromising neurological status. They emphasized that choosing the best treatment approach involves considering a complex set of competing factors that affect various aspects of the patient's outcome. They further emphasized that, with the evolution of newer treatment modalities such as the gamma knife and the auditory brain-stem implant (ABI), the balance between the competing factors that determine the optimal strategy is continually changing. Furthermore, the risks and outcomes of any particular option might be only partly realized at the time of treatment and partly realized some time after the treatment decision. They cited the example of conservative management of a small tumour increasing the chances of preserving hearing longer, but possibly increasing the risks to the facial nerve if surgery is required in the future. A further example of the temporal factor which they described relates to the use of the gamma knife. The incidence of hearing loss with the gamma knife is approximately 50%, but it often occurs in a delayed fashion, allowing more time for the learning of non-auditory methods of communication. However, previous irradiation with the gamma knife, although not an absolute contraindication to the ABI, is thought to be associated with a less good outcome.

Bance and Ramsden advised that the primary goal of management is always to avoid or anticipate life-threatening events. They recommended careful regular clinical assessment coupled with MRI of the neural axis to warn of impending complications and to suggest when surgery is indicated. They suggested that the approach to surgery should be based on a minimal interventionist philosophy and that surgery might be indicated if there is evidence of brain-stem compression or elevated intracranial pressure. The mere presence of tumour in the posterior fossa is not an indication for surgery. If surgery is necessary, total tumour removal should not always be seen as the essential objective, the avoidance of neurological damage being more important. They recommended a similar approach to the management of spinal tumours, which may threaten to cause paraplegia or bladder problems, and may be of more immediate importance than the intracranial tumours.

Bance and Ramsden underlined the importance of avoiding facial nerve damage: this is greatly heightened in NF2 because of the presence of bilateral vestibular Schwannomas, and the terrible burden of bilateral facial weakness. They also drew attention to the potential threat to vision caused by the loss of tearing and the blink reflex, and pointed out that the eyes might already have reduced sensation because of trigeminal nerve involvement by a vestibular Schwannoma, or a separate trigeminal tumour. They advised that the integrity of facial function should be a paramount consideration during surgery for a vestibular Schwannoma, and its function should not be compromised by heroic efforts to remove every last fragment of tumour from the facial nerve.

The subject of hearing preservation is described by Bance and Ramsden as one of the most difficult areas of management of NF2. They state that the total removal of bilateral tumours with preservation of hearing in one or both ears is rarely achieved. They point out that in NF2 there are unique anatomical factors that mitigate against hearing preservation. Although usually arising on the vestibular division of the vestibulocochlear nerve, NF2 tumours tend to invade the cochlear nerve so that the plane of separation between the two is often impossible to define. Furthermore, NF2 tumours are often multicentric in nature and might envelop the cochlear nerve so that the nerve fibres appear to run through the tumour. In such a situation an intracapsular subtotal removal with the aim of hearing preservation would have a high likelihood of failure.

Bance and Ramsden describe the clinical management problem posed by a small vestibular tumour where there is no hearing. They suggest that a case might be made for removal of such a tumour at an early stage, so that the cochlear nerve could be retained and with it the possibility of an eventual cochlear implant. Cochlear implantation has been successfully performed by the authors in this situation.

They also discuss the gamma knife as an alternative to microsurgical removal of vestibular Schwannomas. However, they state their concern regarding significant morbidity to the hearing, both immediately and over time, and to the facial and trigeminal nerves. They refer to the reported risk of hydrocephalus and a fear of inducing malignant change in a hitherto benign tumour. Bance and Ramsden suggest that the gamma knife might have a role in the management of NF2, perhaps in the case of a growing tumour in the only hearing ear, or in patients unfit for conventional microsurgery, or because of the patient's stated preference. However their more recent experience of tumour control following gamma knife treatment in NF2 patients has been discouraging.

Auditory brain-stem implants

NF2 has typically resulted in total deafness after surgical removal of bilateral vestibular Schwannomas. Because of the loss of continuity in the cochlear nerve after tumour removal, cochlear implants are ineffective for this type of deafness. The ABI, based on cochlear implant technology, is a device implanted into the lateral recess of the fourth ventricle to stimulate the cochlear nucleus complex. The ABI has been used since 1979 to provide some auditory sensations to patients deafened after the removal of bilateral vestibular Schwannomas (Hitselberger et al., 1984). The first ABI, which was a single-channel device, was inserted into such a patient at the House Ear Institute, Los Angeles. The ABI stimulates the cochlear nucleus directly, and early results indicate an ability to hear environmental noise and to discriminate pitch differences. The ABI is also reported to enhance lip-reading skills, and some patients will achieve a degree of open-set speech discrimination. The ABI is now considered part of the auditory rehabilitation programme in patients who have total deafness with loss of both cochlear nerves (Laszig et al., 1993). A new generation of multichannel ABI devices has been developed to provide differentiated channels of stimulation (Laszig et al., 1991; Brackmann et al., 1993).

Nevison et al. (2002) reported on the results from a European clinical investigation of the Nucleus multichannel ABI. The objective of their study was to investigate the perceptual benefits and potential risks of implanting the Nucleus multichannel ABI. A total of 27 subjects received a Nucleus 20- or 21-channel ABI between September 1992 and October 1997. All individuals involved in the study had bilateral vestibular Schwannomas. The study used each subject as their own control without a preoperative baseline because residual hearing, if present, was destroyed at surgery by tumour removal. A battery of speech tests was conducted to evaluate each patient's performance and communication abilities. Where possible tests were conducted in the auditory-only, visual-only and auditory–visual conditions at 3 days postoperatively (baseline), at 3-month intervals for the first year and every 12 months thereafter. A subjective performance questionnaire was administered together with an extensive neurological examination at each test interval. The results of the study showed that all 27 subjects involved were successfully implanted with a Nucleus ABI. One subject died 2 days after surgery as the result of a pulmonary embolism unrelated to the device.

Twenty-six subjects underwent device activation and all but one patient received auditory sensation at initial stimulation (96.2%). On average 8.6 (SD ±4.2) of the 21 available electrodes were used in the patients' maps. Performance evaluation measures showed that most users had access to auditory information such as environmental sound awareness, together with stress and rhythm cues in speech that assist with lip-reading. Although most subjects did not achieve any functional auditory-alone, open-set speech understanding, two subjects from the study (7.4%) did receive sufficient benefit to be able to use the ABI in conversation without lip-reading. The authors concluded that, although the medical risks and surgical complexity associated with ABI device implantation are far greater than those for a cochlear implant, the clinical results from their study showed that the Nucleus multichannel ABI was capable of providing a significant patient benefit over risk ratio for subjects suffering loss of hearing due to bilateral vestibular Schwannomas.

Radiosurgery for bilateral vestibular Schwannomas

Radiosurgery has been proposed as an alternative to microsurgical removal of vestibular Schwannomas. Bance and Ramsden (1999) discussed their concerns relating to this treatment modality (see 'Management and treatment of NF2' above).

The International Classification of Functioning, Disability and Health

In 2001, the World Health Organization introduced the latest concepts of the impact of health conditions on individuals in the International Classification of Functioning, Disability and Health (ICF – WHO, 2001). In this classification the positive rather than the negative components of a condition were emphasized, with two-way interactions rather than a simple right-to-left progression. The influence of contextual factors was taken into account. The framework of the ICF 2001 is detailed in Chapter 3.

Psychosocial aspects

There is no published literature regarding the specific psychosocial impacts of NF2 on the affected individual and family. Bateman et al. (2000) reported on the measurements of patients' health-related quality of life (HRQL) following surgery for a unilateral vestibular Schwannoma. Owen et al. (2001) drew attention to the fact that advanced head and neck cancer and its treatment can affect some of the most fundamental and noticeable aspects of life, which may then have a dramatic psychosocial impact on the individual. Wiggins et al. (1992) and Hayes (1992) reported on the psychosocial consequences of predictive testing for Huntington's disease, an incurable transmitted condition. These four publications are reviewed here in the light of how they could relate to individuals with NF2. Ramsden (personal communication, 2003) has emphasized the different psychological impacts on a newly diagnosed NF2 patient, depending on whether he or she has a family history of the condition or is the first family member to be affected.

Bateman et al. (2000) reported that measurements of the patients' HRQL following surgery for a unilateral vestibular Schwannoma was important because patients often present with very mild symptoms, and surgery can impose significant symptoms postoperatively. Studies on HRQL provide structured information from the patients' viewpoint. The study described the most common problems experienced by the patients, using an open-ended questionnaire. The authors pointed out that previous studies on HRQL regarding vestibular Schwannoma surgery had used closed-ended questionnaires, which do not allow the patient to respond freely, but rather ask the patient to respond in a predetermined way. Many questions of the closed-ended type have simple 'yes ' or 'no' answers or responses organized on a scale. The authors argue that this type of closed response format does not allow patients to have their say, and can lead to an inaccurate view of the patients' HRQL, as existing outcome measures tend to be based on the problems perceived as most problematic by healthcare professionals. The advantage of the open-ended questionnaire is that it allows patients to volunteer problems themselves, and is therefore likely to be more representative of what they actually experience by the patients. The questionnaire sent out by the authors asked the patients to:

> Tell us the areas or activities of your life which have been affected by your vestibular Schwannoma operation. Write them down in order of importance, starting with the most important. Please write down as many as you can think of.

This format was similar to that used by Barcham and Stephens (1980). Open-ended questionnaires were sent to 70 consecutive patients who had undergone surgery for a vestibular Schwannoma. As the purpose of their study was to assess the impact of surgery on patients' quality of life, irrespective of immediate or short-term complications, the time following surgery was at least 1 year (range 1-3 years). The patients were aged from 25 to 76 years, with a mean of 49 years. Fifty-three patients out of the 70 returned questionnaires, a response rate of 76%. Patient responses were classified as impairment, disability and handicap, according to the WHO classification. In order to give a general picture of the number of patients reporting problems in specific areas, the responses were grouped into nine categories of functional deficit: auditory dysfunction; eye problems; vestibular problems; psychosocial problems; facial nerve and eating; physical problems (e.g. headache); life skills (e.g. employment); motor problems; and cognitive problems.

The open-ended questionnaire revealed that, after surgery for a vestibular Schwannoma, patients have a wide variety of symptoms. Considering 'functional deficit' patients most commonly reported problems relating to auditory dysfunction. The next most common grouping of symptoms was vestibular dysfunction and eye problems. Psychosocial morbidity was found to be significant in the authors' series. Thirty-four per cent of patients reported a variety of related symptoms such as depression, anxiety and loss of confidence. The authors suggested that, for some patients, early involvement of a clinical psychologist could be useful. Facial nerve and eating difficulties were reported by 32% of the patients. Tinnitus seemed to have a very small impact on patients' lives, being reported in 4% of the authors' series (5 out of 141 responses). Bateman et al. (2000) commented that this was in marked contrast to the incidence of tinnitus found in studies using closed-ended questionnaires.

The authors concluded that the use of open-ended questionnaires provides the most common and important problems as experienced by the patients, rather than suggested by the surgeons and other healthcare professionals. They drew attention to the fact that there were a number of important differences obtained in the study compared with the literature which is based on closed-ended questionnaires. Bateman et al. (2000) reported that with their use of open-ended questionnaires they found that the relative importance of visual and psychosocial symptoms had been highlighted, whereas it appeared that tinnitus was a relatively minor problem. The use of open-ended questionnaires would be expected to allow individuals with NF2 the opportunity to volunteer the problems that they themselves feel to be most significant.

The question of disfigurement following treatment for head and neck cancer and the resulting psychosocial impact was reviewed by Owen et al. (2001). They point out that it has been suggested that patients are particularly vulnerable to psychosocial problems following treatment because social interaction and emotional expression greatly depend on the structure and functional integrity of the head and neck region (Breitbart and Holland, 1988). They advise that it is incumbent upon those involved in the management of patients with advanced head and neck cancer to focus their attentions on quality-of-life improvement, assessment and audit. In NF2, the possibility of the impact of unilateral or bilateral facial paralysis has to be considered, with the resultant psychosocial effects.

Wiggins et al. (1992) and Hayes (1992) discuss the psychological consequences of Huntington's disease, which is also a dominantly transmitted genetic condition with a lethal outcome. Wiggins et al. concluded that predictive testing had potential benefits for the psychological health of people who receive results that indicate either an increase or a decrease in the risk of inheriting the gene for the disease. Hayes gave a personal insight, as an 'at-risk' individual. She recommended that the test should be approached by all parties with the utmost caution, and that it should not be undertaken without safeguards. She stated that for most individuals an answer helps, by eliminating the daily worrying and by allowing time for planning. She urged more open communication among medical professionals, families and volunteer organizations, which can serve as a bridge between the other two groups. Presymptomatic DNA diagnosis can be undertaken in NF2 using molecular genetic techniques. The impact of the diagnosis of NF2 on the presymptomatic individual should be considered.

Ramsden (personal communication, 2003) has emphasized the different psychological impacts on a newly diagnosed NF2 patient, depending on whether he or she has a family history of the condition or is the first family member to be affected. Those who have had a parent with the condition have grown up in the shadow of NF2 and may in part be prepared for the unwelcome diagnosis. For the new mutant, perhaps an apparently fit teenager or young adult with minimal symptoms, the shock is immense. Not only do they have to face the prospect of a shortened life expectancy, total hearing loss and possible disfigurement but they suddenly have to come to terms with the fact that their own children, either already born or in the future, may also have the condition. This is an enormous blow to have to accept. The skill, sensitivity and compassion of the NF2 team, which should include an experienced counsellor, is vital in the ongoing management of the patient and family affected with NF2.

References

Bance M, Ramsden RT (1999) Management of neurofibromatosis type 2. Ear, Nose, and Throat Journal 78: 91–96.

Barcham LJ, Stephens SDG (1980) The use of an open-ended problems questionnaire in auditory rehabilitation. British Journal of Audiology 14: 49–54.

Barker V, Wright E, Nguyen K et al. (1987) Gene for von Recklinghausen neurofibromatosis is in the pericentromeric region of chromosome 17. Science 236: 1100–1102.

Baser ME, Friedman JM, Wallace AJ et al. (2002a) Evaluation of clinical diagnostic criteria for neurofibromatosis 2. Neurology 59: 1759–1765.

Baser ME, Friedman JM, Aeschliman D et al. (2002b) Predictors of the risk of mortality in neurofibromatosis 2. American Journal of Human Genetics 71: 715–723.

Bateman N, Nikolopoulos TP, Robinson K, O'Donoghue GM (2000) Impairments, disabilities, and handicaps after acoustic neuroma surgery. Clinical Otolaryngology 25: 62–65.

Bourn D, Carter SA, Mason S, Evans DGR, Strachan T (1994) Germline mutations in the neurofibromatosis type 2 tumour suppressor gene. Human Molecular Genetics 3: 813–816.

Brackmann DE, Hitselberger WE, Nelson RA et al. (1993) Auditory brainstem implant: 1. Issues in surgical implantation. Otolaryngology – Head and Neck Surgery 108: 624–633.

Breitbart W, Holland J (1988) Psychological aspects of head and neck cancer. Seminars in Oncology 15: 61–69.

Crowe FW, Schull WJ, Neel JV (1956) A Clinical, Pathological and Genetic Study of Multiple Neurofibromatosis. Charles C Thomas, Springfield, IL, p. 15.

Cushing H (1917) Tumors of the Nervus Acousticus and the Syndrome of the Cerebellopontile Angle. Saunders, Philadelphia, PA.

Evans DGR, Birch JM, Ramsden RT (1999) Paediatric presentation of type 2 neurofibromatosis. Archives of Disease in Childhood 81: 496–499.

Evans DGR, Huson SM, Donnai D et al. (1992a) A clinical study of type 2 neurofibromatosis. Quarterly Journal of Medicine 84(304): 603–618.

Evans DGR, Huson SM, Donnai D et al. (1992b) A genetic study of type 2 neurofibromatosis in the United Kingdom. II. Guidelines for genetic counselling. Journal of Medical Genetics 29: 847–852.

Evans DGR, Huson SM, Donnai D et al. (1992c) A genetic study of type 2 neurofibromatosis in the United Kingdom. I. Prevalence, mutation rate, fitness and confirmation of maternal transmission effect on severity. Journal of Medical Genetics 29: 841–846.

Evans DGR, Ramsden R, Huson SM et al. (1993) Type 2 neurofibromatosis: the need for supraregional care? Journal of Laryngology and Otology 107: 401–406.

Evans DGR, Bourn D, Wallace A et al. (1995) Diagnostic issues in a family with late onset type 2 neurofibromatosis. Journal of Medical Genetics 32: 470–474.

Fraser JS (1921) Acoustic tumours of the eighth nerve. Journal of Laryngology and Otology 36: 349–354.

Gardner WJ, Frazier CH (1930) Bilateral acoustic neurofibromas. A clinical study and field survey of a family of five generations with bilateral deafness in thirty-eight members. Archives of Neurology and Psychiatry 23: 266–302.

Gardner WJ, Turner O (1940) Bilateral acoustic neurofibromas. Further clinical and pathologic data on hereditary deafness and Recklinghausen's disease. Archives of Neurology and Psychiatry 4: 76–99.

Gutmann DH, Aylsworth A, Carey JC et al. (1997) The diagnostic evaluation and multidisciplinary management of neurofibromatosis 1 and neurofibromatosis 2. JAMA 278: 51–57.

Hayes CV (1992) Genetic testing for Huntington's disease – a family issue. (Editorial.) New England Journal of Medicine 327: 1449–1451.

Henschen F (1910) Über Geschwülste der hinteren Schädelgrube, insbesondere des Kleinhirnbrückenwinkels. Jena (in German). Gustav Fischer Verlag, Stuttgart, Germany, pp. 283.

Henschen F (1915) Zur Histologie und Pathogenese der Kleinhirnbrücken – winkeltumoren. Archives of Psychiatry 56: 21.

Hitselberger WE, House WF, Edgerton BJ, Whitaker S (1984) Cochlear nucleus implants. Otolaryngology – Head and Neck Surgery 92: 52–54.

Huson SM, Compston DAS, Harper PS (1989) A genetic study of von Recklinghausen neurofibromatosis (NF1) in south east Wales. 1: prevalence, fitness, mutation rate and effect of parental transmission on severity. Journal of Medical Genetics 26: 704–711.

Kanter WR, Eldridge R, Fabricant R, Allen JC, Koerber T (1980) Central neurofibromatosis with bilateral acoustic neuroma: genetic, clinical and biochemical distinctions from peripheral neurofibromatosis. Neurology 30: 851–859.

Laszig R, Kuzma JA, Seifert V, Lehnhardt E (1991) The Hannover auditory brainstem implant: a multiple-electrode prosthesis. European Archives of Oto-Rhino-Laryngology 248: 420–421.

Laszig R, Sollmann WP, Lehnhardt E, Kuzma J (1993) The Nucleus multielectrode auditory brainstem implant - the Hannover model and first results. Paper read at 3rd International Cochlear Implant Conference, 4–7 April 1993, Innsbruck, Austria.

MacCollin M, Mautner VF (1998) The diagnosis and management of neurofibromatosis 2 in childhood. Seminars in Pediatric Neurology 5: 243–252.

MacCollin M, Ramesh V, Jacoby LB et al. (1994) Mutational analysis of patients with neurofibromatosis 2. Americal Journal of Human Genetics 55: 314–320.

Martuza RL, Eldridge R (1988) Neurofibromatosis type 2 (bilateral acoustic neurofibromatosis). New England Journal of Medicine 318: 684–688.

Mautner VF, Lindenau M, Baser ME et al. (1996) The neuroimaging and clinical spectrum of neurofibromatosis 2. Neurosurgery 38: 881–885.

Merel P, Hoang-Xuan K, Sanson M et al. (1995) Predominant occurrence of somatic mutations of the NF2 gene in meningiomas and Schwannomas. Genes Chromosomes Cancer 13: 211–216.

Narod SA, Parry DM, Parboosingh J et al. (1992) Neurofibromatosis type 2 appears to be a genetically homogenous disease. American Journal of Human Genetics 51: 486–496.

National Institutes of Health (1987) Consensus Development Conference Statement on Neurofibromatosis. Neurofibromatosis Research Newsletter 3: 3–6.

National Institutes of Health (1994) Consensus Development Conference Statement on Acoustic Neuroma: December 11–13, 1991. Archives of Neurology 51: 201–207.

National Institutes of Health Consensus Development Conference (1988) Neurofibromatosis Conference Statement. Archives of Neurology 45: 575–578.

Neary WJ, Newton VE, Vidler M et al. (1993) A clinical, genetic and audiological study of patients and families with bilateral acoustic neufibromatosis. Journal of Laryngology and Otology 107: 6–11.

Nevison B, Laszig R, Sollmann W-P et al. (2002) Results from a European clinical investigation of the Nucleus® multichannel auditory brainstem implant. Ear and Hearing 23: 170–183.

Owen C, Watkinson JC, Pracy P, Glaholm J (2001) The psychological impact of head and neck cancer. (Editorial). Clinical Otolaryngology 26: 351–356.

Parry DM, Eldridge R, Kaiser-Kupfer MI et al. (1994) Neurofibromatosis 2 (NF2): clinical characteristics of 63 affected individuals and clinical evidence for heterogeneity. American Journal of Medial Genetics 52: 450–461.

Parry DM, MacCollin MM, Kaiser-Kupfer MI et al. (1996) Germline mutations in the neurofibromatosis 2 gene: correlations with disease severity and retinal abnormalities. American Journal of Human Genetics 59: 529–539.

Recklinghausen F von (1882) Ueber die multiplen Fibrome der haut und ihre Beziehung zu den multiplen Neuromen (in German). Hirschwald, Berlin.

Rouleau GA, Wertelecki W, Haines JL et al. (1987) Genetic linkage of bilateral acoustic neurofibromatosis to a DNA marker on chromosome 22. Nature 329: 246–248.

Rouleau GA, Seizinger BR, Wertelecki W et al. (1990) Flanking markers bracket the neurofibromatosis type 2 (NF2) gene on chromosome 22. American Journal of Human Genetics 46: 323–328.

Rouleau GA, Merel P, Lutchman M et al. (1993) Alteration in a new gene encoding a putative membrane-organising protein causes neurofibromatosis type 2. Nature 363: 515–521.

Ruttledge MH, Narod SA, Dumanski JP et al. (1993) Presymptomatic diagnosis for neurofi-bromatosis 2 with chromosome 22 markers. Neurology 43: 1753-1760.

Ruttledge MH, Andermann AA, Phelan CM et al. (1996) Type of mutation in the neurofi-bromatosis type 2 gene (NF2) frequently determines severity of disease. American Journal of Human Genetics 59: 331-342.

Sato N, Funayama N, Nagafuchi A, Yonemura S, Tsukita S (1992) A gene family consisting of ezrin, radixin and moesin. Its specific localization at action filament/plasma membrane association sites. Journal of Cell Science 103: 131-143.

Seizinger BR, Martuza RL, Gusella JF (1986) Loss of genes on chromosome 22 in tumori-genesis of human acoustic neuroma. Nature 322: 644-647.

Seizinger BR, Rouleau GA, Ozelius LJ et al. (1987a) Genetic linkage of von Recklinghausen neurofibromatosis to the nerve growth factor receptor gene. Cell 49: 589-594.

Seizinger BR, Rouleau G, Ozelius LJ et al. (1987b) Common pathogenic mechanism for three tumor types in bilateral acoustic neurofibromatosis. Science 236: 317-319.

Trofatter JA, MacCollin MM, Rutter JL et al. (1993) A novel moesin-, ezrin-, radixin-like gene is a candidate for the neurofibromatosis 2 tumor suppressor. Cell 72: 791-800.

Welling DB, Glasscock ME (1992) The diagnostic work-up of acoustic neuromas. In: Proceedings of the First International Conference on Acoustic Neuroma, 1992, Copenhagen, Denmark. Kugler, Amsterdam, pp. 101-105.

Wertelecki W, Rouleau GA, Superneau DW et al. (1988) Neurofibromatosis 2: clinical and DNA linkage studies of a large kindred. New England Journal of Medicine 319: 278-283.

WHO (2001) International Classification of Functioning, Disability and Health - ICF. World Health Organisation, Geneva, Switzerland.

Wiggins S, Whyte P, Huggins M et al. (1992) The psychological consequences of predic-tive testing for Huntington's disease. New England Journal of Medicine 327: 1401-1405.

Wishart JH (1822) Case of tumours in the skull, dura mater and brain. Edinburgh Medical Surgical Journal 18: 393-397.

Wolff RK, Frazer KA, Jackler RK et al. (1992) Analysis of chromosome 22 deletions in neu-rofibromatosis type 2-related tumors. American Journal of Human Genetics 51: 478-485.

Young DF, Eldridge R, Gardner WJ (1970) Bilateral acoustic neuroma in a large kindred. JAMA 214: 347-353.

Zucman-Rossi J, Legoix P, Der Sarkissian H et al. (1998) NF2 gene in neurofibromatosis type 2 patients. Human Molecular Genetics 7: 2095-2101.

CHAPTER 11
Moving forward: a life of changes

PATRICIA LAGO-AVERY

When I was 22 years old, studying at Central Michigan University for my bachelor's degree in communication disorders, I discovered a book called *The Psychology of Deafness* by Helmer Myklebust. I was intrigued by the title of this book because it had never occurred to me that there was such a thing as a psychology of deafness. Since I had become profoundly deaf by the age of 21 I decided this book might help me in a quest to understand myself as a deaf person. I had yet to find out I was going blind. So I set about the task of reading the book from front to back, only to wind up totally dismayed by the concepts put forth by the author. It did not take me long to decide that I did not believe in the psychology of deafness. Thirty-one years later, I have read hundreds of books in the field of deafness, psychology, counselling and deafblindness, and I still believe that there is no psychology of deafness or deafblindness for that matter.

What I know is that each of us accumulates experiences throughout our lives, both negative and positive. How we interpret and act upon these experiences is influenced by the many facets of our personality as well as our life circumstances.

I wish to share the story of my life and experiences as an individual who became deafblind as the result of having Usher syndrome type 2A. It is my story and my story alone. Ask any 100 people with Usher syndrome type 2A to tell their life's story, and each story will be very different, from both physiological and psychosocial perspectives. Two or more children with Usher syndrome type 2A within the same family may differ significantly in how they view the world and their place in it, and how they respond to life's challenges.

Background information

Before I share my story as a deafblind person I will explain how deafblindness is defined in the United States, and also provide some information about my family and educational background.

What is deafblindness?

In the United States one can find various definitions of deafblindness. However, the two definitions that are widely used are those defined in the Individual with Disability Educational Act (1990 IDEA, Sec. 622) for educational purposes or the Helen Keller National Center Act (2000, 29 USDS 1905 et seq.) for youths and adults who need additional services beyond the 12th grade of schooling. In the book *Understanding Usher syndrome: introduction for school counselors* (DePietro, 2002), deafblindness is defined as follows:

> a person with any degree of hearing loss combined with vision loss, which interferes with communication, and acquisition of information is considered 'deafblind' even though a person may still have some useful vision and hearing.

What is Usher syndrome?

Usher syndrome is an inherited condition involving hearing loss and retinitis pigmentosa (RP), an eye disorder that gradually causes loss of vision. Researchers have identified three different types of Usher syndrome. The type that I have is characterized by being born with moderate–severe hearing loss and normal balance, with first symptoms of RP showing up in late childhood to early teens. Many individuals with Usher syndrome type 2 do not show severe RP stages until their late thirties or early forties.

Place of my birth and growing-up years

I was born and raised in Bay City, Michigan, on the shores of Lake Huron. Both of my parents are the second from the youngest of eight children in each of their families. My parents met after my father returned from World War II, where he served in the First Infantry Division of the US Army in the European theatre. My mother was working in a factory that produced goods for the war effort. I have two older sisters, the second of whom also has Usher syndrome type 2A. When my second sister was 8 years old and I was 6 years old our parents discovered that we were both hard-of-hearing. We were fitted with hearing aids and sent to the Michigan School for the Deaf for 6 weeks to learn how to use them and go through some evaluations. It was determined that our educational needs would be best met in our home town by attending regular public schools. Both my sister and I attended the public school systems from kindergarten through the 12th grade without any special services other than some speech therapy. After high school I attended a community college and later transferred to a 4-year university, again attending classes with hearing peers without any special services. During these years I experienced two major changes in my hearing: at the age of 15 it dropped from a moderate loss to severe and then at the age of 21 it dropped again to the category of profound deafness.

Adult years

I learned that I had Usher syndrome when working on a research paper for my graduate course in hereditary deafness. Each student was required to pick a topic to research and I chose the topic of Usher syndrome. It was through my research that I started to see some parallels in the symptoms described for Usher syndrome and what I was experiencing with my vision. For example, I could not see in the dark nor could I see objects on the floor. My visual field was shrinking. Another example is demonstrated by the following story:

> One day I was bending over to pick something up off the floor. I did not see that a wooden chair was right next to me. I hit the back of the chair with my face and broke one of my front teeth. The downside is that I lost one of my front teeth but the cap on that tooth actually looks better than the old tooth.

When later it was verified that indeed I did have Usher syndrome, it was quite a shock. At that time, my vision was still in what is called the mild stages of RP. I was 24 years old and nearing the completion of my bachelor's degree, applying to graduate school and getting ready to move on to a new life at the University of Arizona in Tucson. I basically decided I did not have time in my life to deal with the diagnosis of Usher syndrome.

After I completed my masters degree in rehabilitation and counselling for the deaf from the University of Arizona I moved to Rochester, New York to accept a position at the National Technical Institute for the Deaf/Rochester Institute of Technology working as a carer and personal counsellor to college-age students who were deaf or hard-of-hearing. During the first 10 years of employment at NTID/RIT I struggled with many issues – professional, personal and medical – as well as trying to deal with continuation of vision and hearing losses due to Usher syndrome. I will elaborate on this later in the chapter.

At the age of 38 I married my husband, Joseph Avery, who is hearing and had been a professional colleague since my arrival at NTID/RIT. He was a widower with four sons. When we married his two older sons were living on their own but I suddenly became a mother to his two younger and very lively boys. In August 2003 Joe and I celebrated our 15th wedding anniversary. As our lives became entwined we faced and met the many challenges of marriage, parenthood and serving dual careers while raising families, not to mention the continuing decline of my vision and hearing.

Losses and gains

What are the losses?

The most important concept to keep in mind is that individuals with Usher syndrome (type 1, 2 or 3), will experience significant losses in their lives. These losses are not only of hearing and vision, but also of independence, employment or career, of friendships, communication with loved ones and former colleagues and of self-identity if one does not have a good support system in place or the personal perseverance to forge ahead. Added are the losses of many things they were able to do but can no longer do alone. Examples of these types of losses are:

- Driving a car: in the USA this is a huge loss because public transportation is not very good except in the larger cities. It impacts everything from going to work, driving to the doctor's office and taking your children to school.
- Riding a bicycle.
- Rock climbing.
- Hiking difficult trails.
- Being able to find clothing in the stores easily or at all. Tunnel vision makes it very difficult to scan the racks for clothing one might like or had seen just minutes before but can no longer locate.

Some of these activities can be continued, with modifications. For example, I still ride on a tandem bicycle with my husband, and we recently invested in a recumbent tricycle that I can ride independently in safe low-traffic areas. I also continue to hike using a trekking pole. But I move slower and with caution on difficult trails. Every task becomes more difficult and therefore requires time, effort and rehabilitation to learn new ways of functioning. Some of this rehabilitation does not require formal training but just trying to figure out for oneself how to continue to have a good quality of life. Other times new skills should be learned and professional help is required.

The years of crisis for me spanned 10 years from the time I found out I had Usher syndrome at the age of 24 until I turned a corner at the age of 34, realizing and accepting that Usher syndrome was a part of my life, my burden to carry but not get me down. The psychological turmoil that I dealt with during those years required many steps in a long hard journey. These were years of depths of depression, growth and, eventually, progressing with the discovery of whom I was as an individual. During this time I also continued to have fun, laughter, friendships and love from my family (parents, sisters and their families). Much of this growth had nothing to do with being deaf and having RP while other areas of growth had everything to do with being deaf and having RP.

As I mentioned earlier, I am an avid reader. But during this 10-year period of time there were three books that stand out very clearly in my mind as books that helped me in the process of moving ahead with my life. The first was a book called *In the Search of Serenity* by Lewis F. Presnall (Presnall, 1958) given to me by a friend in graduate school. The book was written for recovering alcoholics, but it is great for anyone who is trying to find their way in life. From this book the major lesson I learned was that I must take one day at a time and enjoy those days and that I needed to learn to accept those things I cannot change. The second book I found while studying for comprehensive exams and it was called *Helplessness: on depression, development and death* by Martin Seligman (Seligman, 1975). This book addressed the issues of how people often become depressed based on how they learn to view themselves in the context of their lives. They learn to feel helplessness, as if they have no control over life events. We do not necessarily have control over illness or other God-given events in our lives, but we do have control over how we choose to respond or deal with what life hands us. The third book, and perhaps the most valuable to me in terms of dealing with losses, was *On Death and Dying* by Elisabeth Kubler-Ross (Kubler-Ross, 1969). In her work with people who were terminally ill, Kubler-Ross noted patterns of coping with the prospect of dying which she described in a stage theory. Patients tended to progress through various stages to the point of being able to accept the termination of life. This theory also has meaning for describing psychological response to serious loss of any kind. Obviously as a person with Usher syndrome, I was not terminally ill or dying although deep in my heart I might have felt that I was emotionally dying from time to time. As I thought about Kubler-Ross's book and the concepts of isolation, denial, anger, bargaining, depression and acceptance as part of the grieving process, mourning for what one once had and no longer has, I was able to modify the model to fit my own situation. And in my situation I was dealing with continuous losses and deterioration of hearing and vision. What I found is that I needed to go through all these stages each time I felt a loss. However, as time went by and the more I experienced additional losses, my recovery period of depression, anger or whatever stage I was in during the process of mourning would become shorter. But, in addition to the physical changes I also had to deal with changes in my self-concept, and how others viewed me and interacted with me. Because I worked in the field of deafness where professionals as well as others seem to need to put labels on people I was often viewed as hard-of-hearing, hard-of-hearing going deaf, hearing-impaired, hearing and visually impaired, deaf and visually impaired or deafblind. As one can imagine, it would be so easy to get confused as to where one might fit in. Fortunately for me I by then had developed a pretty strong core of whom I was. And it was obvious to me that I was Patti and always have been Patti. So much of me had nothing to do with my vision and hearing losses. Coming to this conclusion has helped me tremendously with keeping my self-identity intact.

During those 10 years I also saw a therapist from time to time. During my darkest days I saw a therapist every 2 weeks for 18 months. It was time well spent to help me heal, grow and move on with my life.

One of the things that people often asked me is 'how did you used to hear and see compared to now?'. When I say 'now', I mean before the cochlear implant which I received six months ago. So I will try to give you some ideas of these changes in my hearing and vision.

Hearing and vision as a young child

I remember hearing the television when my parents first got a set in 1955. I was 5 years old and still had not been diagnosed with a hearing loss. However, I had to sit very close to the TV to hear and understand what was being said. My parents thought I was near-sighted and had me tested. Sure enough, I needed glasses. But I still sat near the TV. One year later I was diagnosed with a bilateral moderate hearing loss, along with my sister. We got fitted with the big body aids used in those days and life then was back to normal. I wore this device every day of my life from the time I got up to the time I went to bed. Sounds were very important to me and I enjoyed hearing everything. I watched TV and understood. I understood my parents, and could talk on the phone when we got our first telephone. I could hear cars in the street when I was riding my bike. I do not remember feeling any different than other kids and do not remember not understanding things in the classroom. My hearing remained reasonably stable until I was 15 years old. Life was good, full of childhood play and school.

Hearing and vision as an adolescent

When I was a freshman in high school I experienced some dizziness and disorientation for about one month. Then, I noticed my hearing had changed. When I was tested it was discovered that my hearing had deteriorated to the level of a severe hearing loss. I received a new hearing aid, and started wearing it in my right ear instead of the left ear because of a recruitment factor (hearing sound uncomfortably loud) in the left ear. But I noticed that I still did not hear as well as before. Understanding in the classroom became a major effort but I was still able to keep up. I could always understand my teachers but not the other students in the back of the room. Before the most recent hearing loss, I could understand everyone in the classroom. Both my pure-tone average and my discrimination level changed. I still continued to talk on the phone but it required more effort. Like most adolescents music had been important in my life, and it continued to be. I still enjoyed music and could understand many of the words. But I know that I started to fall behind in my vocabulary because I was not hearing new words or their pronunciations as well as before.

The only subconscious awareness I had regarding my vision was noticing that I could not see well at night. But I figured this was true of others as well. After all, it is dark out there! My social life changed somewhat during these years. I did not function well in large-group interactions. My friendships changed as well, but I continued to have a couple of close friendships with two girlfriends from high-school years that continue to this day. I also had a steady boyfriend for 3 years.

Hearing and vision as a young adult

At the age of 21 when I was a junior in college, I experienced the second significant change in my hearing. This is when I feel I left the hearing world and started moving more to being deaf. My hearing dropped to a profound hearing loss. I was no longer able to carry on phone conversations competently although I did continue to try with my parents. At the age of 27, I finally said no more phone conversations. That is when my family and I started to use the teletype to communicate and keep in touch. It was also at this time in my life (aged 21–23 years) that I became very confused about my career goals. As I became profoundly deaf, I felt my career options were slipping away. Also I faced some memorable acts of discrimination and very poor advice from teachers and other concerned professionals who were counselling me to go into science and mathematics and not into careers that involved working with people. One example of discrimination I experience is best told by the following story:

I was nearing the end of my senior year. During my last semester I was taking two graduate-level courses. One was in counselling. I loved this course and felt I had the desire and potential to work in the helping field. I had decided I wanted to be a counsellor and work with deaf and hard-of-hearing students. I arranged to visit the Michigan School for the Deaf and interview a man who was a counsellor there. He was very blunt and told me he did not know of one successful deaf counsellor and did not encourage my endeavours. As a matter of fact I was told that I would find it very difficult trying to deal with the hearing world on a professional level. Fortunately by then I had developed more self-confidence and decided he was a person who was not very supportive of deaf people.

My ability to clearly hear voices in everyday speech continued. The voices, yes, but my discrimination ability was severely compromised. However, with my lip-reading skills I could still converse easily with hearing people, both those I knew and those I did not know. I could no longer understand words in songs to music, but if I had the words written in front of me I could follow along with the music. I could still recognize individual voices of friends and family members, but I was becoming more dependent on lip-reading and sign language. Having those two skills, plus moving from a total hearing world to working and being with deaf and hard-of-hearing people were blessings. Having sign language in my life is very important and will continue to be very important. Some day I will need to depend on tactile communication, and one cannot use tactile communication unless one knows sign language. I could still hear the phone ring. I heard most sounds in the environment, an ability that helped me feel safe – even more so when, at the age of 24, I learned that I had Usher syndrome. As my vision deteriorated, my ability to hear environmental sounds, and to be able to recognize people's voices in professional meetings, helped me tremendously in the area of communication and staying in touch with the world.

Although I learned about my vision at the age of 24 during the last month of my undergraduate studies I was not ready to deal with it. I basically ignored this information and focused on finishing my degree, applying to graduate schools and finding a job to support myself for the next 6 months.

I asked one of my professors at Central Michigan University about Usher syndrome but he did not know much about it and I never told him I had the condition. It was not until after I started graduate school in Arizona that I really started to think about Usher syndrome and do research in the medical school library. Through the process of researching I also discovered that my older sister might also have this condition. I became depressed and distraught. My depression was mostly due to learning I was going blind and that my sister might have this condition as well. My parents did not know anything about Usher syndrome. My doctor in Michigan just told me I had RP; he himself was not aware of the condition of Usher syndrome. The only other thought I had was whether this genetic condition could be passed on to any children I might have. I did my research in this area as well and concluded that most likely if I had children they would not have the condition unless the father also had Usher syndrome, but they would be carriers. Even though I was new to Arizona and did not know anyone there I decided to take a chance and speak to my program chairperson, Dr Larry Stewart. He was a deaf man who I felt might be able to answer some of my questions. He also was a clinical psychologist. Larry, as I began to call him after I became a professional colleague in the field of deafness and counselling, was the perfect person with whom to speak. He soon grasped my dilemma, my emotional state of mind and also my ignorance of my condition even though I was conducting research. The problem was that there seemed to be very little information about Usher syndrome back in 1975, and some of the information was inaccurate. What frightened me the most was reading about patients who had Usher syndrome and were also psychotic. My imagination began to go wild with this knowledge. Larry quickly assured me that these articles were written about patients who were both mentally ill and had Usher syndrome; it did not mean that everyone with Usher syndrome was or would become mentally ill. However, I told him I could easily understand how one might become mentally ill if they did not understand what was happening. Larry referred me to a retinal specialist as I had never talked with a doctor thoroughly about my vision. So during the first year of my graduate studies I dealt not only with living in a new place 3000 miles from my family and friends but also trying to come to terms with my Usher syndrome. I was able to lift myself out of the depression with help from Dr Stewart, new friends and reading books about the human spirit and trying to understand the psychology of losses. By the time I finished graduate work and left for an internship at NTID/RIT I was feeling mentally strong again and ready to take on the world and new experiences. I basically decided that I could not change having Usher syndrome but I could learn to take one day at a time. I could embrace whatever life had to give me and I would drink in all I could see as long as possible. And I made sure I never closed my eyes while travelling by car because I never wanted to miss anything!

Hearing and vision in my thirties and forties

Even though my hearing loss changed from severe to profound at the age of 21, my discrimination ability with use of the hearing aid continued to be about 75% in quiet places, quiet being the key word. This continued until my late twenties. As I became older my discrimination ability changed very slowly, but by the time I was 40 my discrimination ability in quiet places was zero so I was depending on sign language, lip-reading and voice recognition more and more as well as my ability to recognize environmental sounds. I was still able to hear the phone ringing, cars on the street and other warning signals. I also still enjoyed music for the most part, but not like a hearing person. I could enjoy instrumental music such as piano, guitar, harp or violin, as well as attending orchestral concerts. Then very slowly I started to lose those abilities and by the time I was 45 I could no longer recognize people I knew by the sound of their voices. Music just became noise, and environmental sounds all became a blur of noise that was unbearable to listen to. I started to watch TV without the sound and would often take my hearing aid off in the evenings because I could no longer tolerate constant noise in my ears and head. I continued to use my hearing aid during the day when at work, or when family and hearing friends were around. These changes of hearing greatly changed the way I functioned as a person. At first I thought my vision was changing because I just did not seem to be in touch with the world as well as before. However, vision testing showed that it had not changed. So the next step was to test my hearing. Pure-tone testing revealed no change, but, again, I had zero discrimination for speech. But the subtle changes that I experienced are not ones that can be measured by an audiologist.

During these years my vision continued to deteriorate from moderate RP to severe RP. I also developed cataracts, which further detracted from my limited vision. Dealing with glare from the sun and snow was a major problem, and I used special glasses to help me with this aspect of my vision. With the losses of more vision I also experienced other losses that accompany vision loss. Loss of not being able to ride my bike independently, loss of giving up my driver's licence, loss of independence in simple everyday life. Living without a car in the USA makes everyday life very difficult unless one lives in a large metropolitan area with good public transportation. I love travelling in Europe because it seems that one can travel anywhere by public transportation. This certainly is not true in the USA where the car is king. I experienced many other losses. I love the outdoors, but I found hiking becoming more difficult. Rock hopping, jumping from rock to rock while crossing streams, was not something I could do anymore. These were years of great losses for me and bouts of depression.

What were the gains?

But these were also years of significant growth, new beginnings and a new life as a married woman and mother. I learned how to change some of the ways I do things to keep me feeling good about myself. I decided I could still ride a bike if my husband and I used a tandem. I could still hike if I used a trekking pole. I go slower than other people, but the positive aspect is my husband gets twice as much exercise because he will hike ahead and then back-track to make sure I am still standing and moving. Using the trekking pole keeps me from falling if I should stumble on a rock or root in the ground. It is like having three legs. Now my focus is on trying to be creative to think of ways to do things I enjoy, but in a different way. I still love to canoe, and that is not a problem. I have learned so many different ways to overcome my disabilities that they are just second nature to me.

At the age of 44 it was decided that I would benefit from cataract surgery and I received lens implants in both eyes. I went into this process with a little nervousness but my surgeon assured me this was a very routine type of surgery and had a 99.9% success rate. I decided I was willing to take the risk and it was well worth it. The surgery was performed in the fall of 1994, first on my right eye and then on my left. What I remember the most about the results of this surgery was the brilliance of the colours of the fall foliage and being able to see the leaves on the top of the trees. It felt like a miracle to me. But the best part of it all was there was no longer any glare when I was outside, or inside in my office or meeting rooms. The strain on my eyes just melted away. This is not to say I did not continue to have eye strain – I did, because of my limited visual field and having to depend on my eyes all day long for understanding people. My career as a counsellor and professor required continuous communication, day in and day out. But I no longer had to deal with the glare issue and my central vision was much clearer.

Probably the biggest and most difficult issues to deal with have been giving up my driver's licence and having to use the cane. Using the cane is an emotional signal that is hard to overcome. It means I can no longer navigate my environment safely. It means that others will know I am blind and some will assume I cannot see anything. It also leaves me feeling more vulnerable. But, as I learned, the cane also can be liberating. It means I do not need to depend on others to lead me. It tells others in my environment to move aside so I do not bump into them. When people see my cane they seem to part like the Red Sea did for Moses. This positive effect was very apparent to me because I worked on a college campus and often had to walk around campus for various meetings. There were always many people to bump into, but they moved out of my way for the cane. When I talk about my cane I tell people that 'the cane is for both them and me'. They seem puzzled by that comment, but I explain that the cane is to keep everyone and me in my environment safe. If they do not pay attention to my cane and run into me, they could seriously hurt themselves as well as me. So at the age of 45 I learned some basic cane skills. Three years later I realized it was time to learn additional skills that would help me function better as a deafblind person, and that meant going to the Helen Keller National Center for Deaf-Blind Youth and Adults (HKNC) on Long Island, New York.

My goals for attending HKNC were:

- To gain more intensive mobility and orientation training.
- To upgrade my computer skills and learn about technology that would help me as my vision deteriorated.
- To learn how to manage and set up my kitchen so that I could work more effectively.
- To learn tactile communication. I already knew sign language so converting that knowledge to tactile was not as hard as I thought it would be.
- To have time for myself to come to terms with all the changes in my life.

The last of my goals was critical because, when you are a wife, a mother and a professional in the helping field, much of your energy goes to others. You really need time away from everything else to focus on yourself, to cry, to laugh and to heal. I was able to do this with three other women at HKNC who had Usher syndrome type 2. Three of us were married with children. One was a young woman from Holland who was thinking about marriage and family. We had a wonderful time together. We shared our life stories, our frustrations with having Usher syndrome but also we laughed at the many common experiences we encountered that to others might not sound very funny. But to us our shared experience helped us to form a bond. I forged new friendships that would stay with me for many years. My only regret is that my stay at HKNC was too short. I returned home after 6 weeks to go back to work and be with my family.

Hearing and vision in the fifties: more gains than losses

I had not given much thought to having a cochlear implant at that point. However, a couple of years later I started to think about this possibility but never expressed these thoughts to anyone else. It would take another 2 years before I started to verbalize these thoughts to Joe. Interestingly enough, he was not very supportive of the idea. Then, by the time I was 50 years old, one of my deaf friends, Sally Skyer, and I started to talk more about this concept. It would take me two more years to conclude that a cochlear implant might be something that would help me keep in touch with my world more effectively. I certainly was not going to get my vision back. I credit my friend Dr Michael Stinson in helping to lead the way as well as some of my former students who have had cochlear implants. Michael's experience with his cochlear implant also had a positive influence on Joe. Since Michael and I had known each other for almost 22 years and have watched each other deal with the challenges of hearing deterioration, he thought that my getting a cochlear implant would mirror his experience. With my husband's full support I started a 3-month process of evaluation in June 2002 and followed with surgery on 17 October 2002. I was connected to my cochlear implant processor on 19 November 2002.

I am now 53 years old. My vision has not changed much in the past 7 years. My hearing has changed dramatically since receiving the cochlear implant. The hearing I have regained has taken me on a journey that I never expected.

Experience as a deafblind person after the cochlear implant

More gains

By now, the reader should have a fairly good idea of how my hearing and vision deteriorated over the years. The following is what I wrote to my family and friends soon after being connected to my cochlear implant.

November 20, 2002

Dear Family and Friends,
Yesterday was my hook-up day, the day Joe and I have been long waiting for. I

know my family and friends also have been waiting for this special day. It was an amazing experience to say the least.

Although I have not been able to understand speech for the past 18 years or more I was able to hear environmental sounds and voices. Up until about 7 years ago I was even able to recognize voices of different people and know who was talking. I also was able to enjoy some music, for example, solo instruments like the piano or guitar, etc. I lost that enjoyment around the age of 45 as well as being able to identify people who were talking by the sound of their voices.

Yesterday I was turned on to my CI at approximately 4:15 p.m. after a series of tests and mapping of the processor. Dr Mark Orlando, my audiologist, mapped my processor with three different programs to try for the next few days until I go back to see him on Friday. The first thing I heard, after the individual tones testing, was Mark's voice. At first it was a shock that I not only heard his voice but I understood what he was saying. Up until that time Joe was interpreting in sign language everything that Mark was saying to me. At first I was not sure if I was understanding Mark because the sound was different but also it seemed weird to me because it was like the words were in my head and I was understanding with my head instead of having the sound go through the hearing aid into my ear and trying to travel to my brain and most of it getting lost along the way. Now it is as if the sound goes into the part of my brain that needs to interpret the sound. But then Mark asked me some questions that required answers from me. I was startled to hear my voice, as it sounded too loud to me. It also did not sound like me. I decided I did not like my voice but then Joe started to talk and although he sounded a little different he did sound like Joe and he has such a nice warm voice. I understood him completely without any work or effort. Wow . . . I started to cry. It was so emotional. I think if I had been alone and allowed to let myself go I would have sobbed. But I held my tears back so that I could continue my work with the audiologist. However one of the things I do not like about what I am hearing is a constant chirpy noise in my head. Mark said this would go away with time (I certainly hope so).

Walking down the hall of the hospital I could hear voices of people who were many feet away. I also realized that I did not hear noises but discrete sounds such as people talking and footsteps on the floor. In the past all I could hear was all the noise that masked over voices.

Driving home in the car:
We left the hospital at 5:30 p.m. and it was after dark. The car engine is loud, and then I hear this blink . . . blink . . . blink sound. At first I did not know what that was but then realized that the noise sounded like how the turn signal looks when it is blinking so sure enough that was what it was. Then Joe started talking to me and I was thinking 'why is he talking to me, he knows I cannot understand and see in the dark?' However everything he was saying was turning into words in my head and I understood him. We only had a very dim faint light on the side of his face from the vanity mirror on my side of the car. At the same time I was listening to the motor of the van: how it sounds when it is idling, how it sounds when he first takes off from a stop light, how it sounds when he is driving along and then he is talking to me some more and I understand everything he is saying. It was not like a major conversation but just him asking me questions and me understanding him so

I could respond. We have never been able to communicate in the dark under any situations in the past. The other thing I noticed is that I am not bothered by noises in the car. Before all the noise from the car would override voices. Now it is like the voice in the car is the dominant sound. We arrived home and from the garage I could hear the dogs barking in the house. Speaking of dogs . . . while I have been typing this up in the study on the second floor the dogs have been barking away in the Florida room which is quite a distance from where I am sitting. I think I could slowly go insane with their barking!!! They are barking at Jim next door who is outside raking up his leaves.

Suppertime with Joe, Jeff our son and Elaine our daughter in law: I understand everything everyone is saying but I still need to use my lip-reading skills with them. Before I could never understand Jeff fully because he is difficult to lip-read. But now with my CI and lip-reading I can understand him about 95% of the time. Later that night we watched TV and I realized that if I am lip-reading the person who is talking on the screen, I can understand what they are saying with my CI and lip-reading skills without watching the captioning. I understand about 50%. That is pretty good compared to 0% before. But then I got tired so I decided to go upstairs and unplug myself and just used captioning with the TV in the bedroom.

(Right now I hear music coming from someplace so I need to go and explore . . . be right back) Yes, Joe was playing on his banjo!

Other sounds I notice:
• Keys clicking when I type.
• When the dogs are eating their treats I hear the crunching noises of the treats they are chewing.
• When I made a light breakfast of toast and peanut butter I heard the following sounds: picking up jar from the Lazy Susan, the jar when I sat it down, the lid when I was taking if off the jar, the smearing sounds of putting peanut butter on the toast, the water gurgling down my throat as I drank it.
• Feet on the tile and wood floors
• Dogs' noises when they are wrestling with each other.
• Water from the different sinks in the house all sound different.
• The dish rag has a sound when I throw it down on the sink.
• I hear the dogs' happy sounds when I am petting them.

Lunch out with Sally the next day:
Heard the door bell ring and dogs barking (have always heard the dogs barking at the door before, though). Her car engine sounds different than our van. Still noticed that I am not bothered by background noises but can hear voices. At the restaurant I hear the waitress's voice and understand her without too much difficulty, however I also hear all these other individual voices in the background. I do not understand what people are saying though but I heard their voices. Before all I heard was awful noise in my ears. The noise is not there now . . . just individual voices.

The rest of the day was just listening to house sounds like the light switches, my walking sounds on the floor, the noise of the dog bone box when I open it, etc. Well that is all I have to report right now.
Love,
Patti

Since I wrote that letter, 8 months have passed. I have learned to enjoy music again. I understand words of songs that I used to hear when I was a teenager. I also often can follow words in new songs if I have the words written in front of me. I am talking on the telephone for the first time since I was in my early twenties. Every week it seems like I have some new experience in hearing that is amazing to me. I feel like my brain is functioning differently. But for the most part my life has become so much easier. I feel more like a person who is blind and has a mild hearing loss when I have my cochlear implant on. Of course when I am sleeping, swimming and doing things that require that I remove the cochlear implant then I am totally deaf again. But this does not bother me because I know I have the option of plugging in my cochlear implant again when I want. I have gone from having zero discrimination ability in my pre-implant audiology testing to 99% understanding of short sentences. I can understand my husband most of the time when he is speaking to me without lip-reading if I am paying attention. I understand most people almost 100% of the time. Once in a while I might have to ask for them to repeat a sentence. What is most amazing is that I do not have any problems understanding people who speak English with a foreign accent. In the past this was almost always a problem for me.

The emotional impact of getting my hearing back has been like being on a roller-coaster. I have talked with a few of my deaf and hard-of-hearing friends who received a cochlear implant and have been very happy with the results. But they have not experienced the extreme emotional highs and lows I have experienced. We have concluded that it must be because as a deafblind person getting so much of my hearing back has enhanced my life in ways that they would not notice for themselves. For example, not hearing ice clinking in a glass of water is no big deal for the deaf person. But for a deafblind person hearing ice clinking in the water glass tells us that someone is there pouring water into our glass. The deaf person can see this, the deafblind person cannot. So hearing this information tells us many things. It helps us be aware that someone is standing next to us, that the water glass is being filled, it tells us not to move while this is happening so we will not bump the server. It also tells us if we want something this is the time to ask the server to help us because we know he or she is at the table. In the past I would have to ask someone else at the table to let me know when the server came and sometimes it would be forgotten. This is just one example of how my hearing has helped me feel more connected with the world. I also feel safer because I can hear sounds in my environment such as a car or bus and understand them. I know this because I used to hear those sounds when I was younger. I did not need to go through rehabilitation to relearn many of the environmental sounds. Had I been born profoundly deaf I would have needed to learn to identify sounds. There are many new sounds in the environment that did not exist when I was a child, like the beeping of the computer and the computer talking to me from time to time. Also my oven, microwave, toaster all beep to let me know they are ready or done. That was very bewildering at first and I needed to ask my husband about those sounds. I love to hear the birds sing, even the sparrows whose songs are not as pretty as other bird songs. It would take pages to explain how much the cochlear implant has enhanced my life. I know the results vary from person to person. But I have spoken with other deafblind people who were born profoundly deaf, received a cochlear implant and are very happy with the results. They are happy because they have learned to understand many environmental sounds that are so important to deafblind people.

The emotional impact of the cochlear implant, as I mentioned before, has been characterized by some extreme highs and some lows. The highs come from the thrill of hearing old sounds and new sounds. The lows come from the realization of how much I have missed in my life when both my hearing and vision were changing. It is hard to put into words, but I never really realized how much work was required to maintain and keep up with my hearing and deaf peers. I just did what was necessary to keep myself productive as a career-oriented individual with a family. I focused on being proactive and trying to solve everyday issues that would keep me on equal footing with my other colleagues. That was my focus. Sometimes I feel flashes of anger with this realization. The anger does not last long. But I hope I never forget how difficult my life used to be. I want to be able to convey that knowledge to others who work in the field of deafblindness. And I want to always remember that each deafblind person has his or her own individual challenges.

But now I mostly just enjoy each day as it comes. This has been my philosophy since I was 25 years old. Take one day at a time, savour and enjoy that day. Learn the lessons of life that each day brings, both the good and the bad. All are valuable in the journey through life.

Conclusions

In concluding my story I want to share what has been my motto throughout most of my adult life. One must prepare for the worst but hope for the best. This is why I chose to learn as many communication methods as possible as well as rehabilitation skills such as mobility and orientation, Braille and independent living skills.

At this point in my life the journey continues. Every day brings new experiences, new frustrations and the intense feeling of being alive. My life is full of laughter, joy, bouts of sadness as well as all the other emotions that come with life's ups and downs. I have managed to keep my sense of humour intact in spite of all I have been through. I am a wife, mother, grandmother, daughter, sister, sister-in-law, aunt, niece, cousin and friend as well as a professional in the field of deafness, counselling and deafblindness. My work involves chairing the Deaf Blind Collaborative Committee in Rochester, New York, serving on the board of directors for the American Association of the Deaf Blind, presenting, writing and publishing nationally and internationally. In addition to all the above, it is a blessing to be able to have contact with many former students from the NTID/RIT who have touched my life throughout the years and taught me much.

References

DePietro LJ (2002) Understanding Usher Syndrome: an introduction for school counselors. Helen Keller National Center for Deaf-Blind Youths and Adults, Sands Point, NY.

Kübler-Ross E (1969) On Death and Dying. Macmillan, New York.

Presnall LP (1958) The Search for Serenity. Utah Alcoholism Foundation, Salt Lake City.

Seligman M (1975) Helplessness: on depression, development and death. Freeman, San Francisco, CA.

CHAPTER 12
My genetic deafness

JILL JONES

I have Treacher Collins syndrome (TCS), a low-prevalence syndrome affecting approximately 1 in 10 000–50 000 births in the general population (NORD, 1999). The condition was first described by Dr Treacher Collins, a British ophthalmologist, in 1846, and his name was linked to the syndrome in 1900. The syndrome is also called mandibular dystosis or first arch syndrome (Gibbin, 1988). It is a condition caused by an autosomal dominant gene, which means that only one parent has to carry the gene for a child to develop the syndrome. It can also result from a 'mutated' gene, occurring randomly and becoming part of the person's genetic code. This is said to be true for 60% of people with TCS.

Physical appearance of people with Treacher Collins syndrome

Those who have the so-called 'treacle gene' responsible for TCS have the classical underdeveloped or misaligned jaws with resulting dental, speech or feeding problems. Breathing can be affected because of the narrowness of breathing passages. Unusually small or malformed ears or absence of external ears and/or canals can be found, as can slanting down of the eyes and notching of the lower eyelids. Some people with TCS may have a growth of scalp hair towards the cheeks. Deafness may or may not be a feature, and is usually conductive, generally with an approximate 60 dB loss. TCS is classed as being a similar type of genetic condition to Goldenhar's syndrome.

As the features of TCS can vary so much from person to person, many people have not been diagnosed because they have only a few symptoms. This was the case for me, as I was not found to have TCS until I was in my mid-40s. Although I have some of the craniofacial characteristics, it was not until two adults with TCS noted our similarity, especially when we sat in a row and compared our profiles, that I definitely knew there was a name for my condition. However, there are some people with TCS who have medical features that call for a tracheostomy or eye operations, or can lead to other clinical intervention.

I was operated on several times through my childhood for cosmetic reasons, to build up the tiny lump of tissue on the left-hand side, and to give me some sort of a pinna on the right, as I had no external ear at all on that side. At the same time, or at different times from the outer ear operations, I had 'corrective surgery' to try to cure my deafness. It now feels more like being treated as a guinea-pig, as nothing happened except to give my parents false hope.

When I look through the medical notes on TCS, I am always struck by the amount of negative language, i.e. 'malformed', 'abnormalities', 'risk', 'defective gene', and even 'bad seed' (Ballantyne, 1970). Being considered a defective person is not good for one's self-esteem, already wavering because of being 'normalized' in mainstream education. It is enough to look in the mirror or to see photographs and videos to see the difference from the so-called 'norm'. I do have the 'look' of TCS, so might be expected, after almost 60 years of knowing this, to have accepted this. To a greater extent I have learnt to live with myself for who I am, but there is still an element of shock when I see myself as others see me. Is this vanity, or is it a sense of grief to know that I am not as feminine as I would like to be, in a society that places so much emphasis on female looks? For the general population, 'look-ism' (an important part of TCS) and 'deaf-ism' often go hand in hand, so that one poor attitude often merges into the other, a hidden discrimination that is just as powerful as other forms of discrimination.

I do not advocate genetic research into TCS, as it is a societal problem, and not ours. It is up to society to change its attitude towards diversity in looks. I fully support a person with gigantism (large head and chin), who has recently received a fair amount of publicity, who will not contemplate having cosmetic surgery. For the same reason I certainly would not.

It is interesting to me that both my children have a few of the features of TCS, one slightly more than the other. Neither of them is deaf. Fortunately I was spared the worry of wondering if they would have TCS, as I was unaware I had the condition during pregnancy, although I was distinctly relieved that their ears were perfectly formed. It is one thing to find an inner peace with respect to look-ism. It is another to want your children to be forced to go through the stages of acceptance as well, maybe never reaching it. When I was diagnosed, my children were too, at the ages of about 12 and 14 years. I have since noted that, like myself, my son produces excessive mucus, and this was a contributing factor in his having to give up professional football. I do not know if I will be fortunate enough to be a grandmother, but if so, I will fully support my children and their partners in going for genetic counselling if they wish to, or with any other support and information.

Hearing and communication

People with TCS are said to have moderate and conductive deafness, usually 60 dB, which means that we are thought to respond well to bone-conduction hearing aids and bone-anchored hearing aids (BAHAs). This may well be so, but we are still deaf and need to have a visual language, so, like all hard-of-hearing children, we should be exposed to sign bilingualism in education. I was offered a BAHA twice by an ENT specialist, but he finally accepted my refusals on the basis that I am a British Sign Language (BSL) user. This was also an acknowledgement of my Deaf identity.

There is much debate about the importance of Deaf identity development. Corker (1996) cites, among others, Kannapel (1994) who suggests that:

> Deaf people's cultural identity is made up of how they view themselves in terms of language identity, personal identity and social identity (which she calls identity types), all of which are strongly interrelated.

Most deaf children are not given 'permission to be Deaf' through childhood, and are taught orally (Jones, 1995). It is essential that all deaf children, regardless of level of hearing loss, are sign bilingual, so that we have a language of identity, a social language and also access to information in mainstream society, i.e. in school, further education and at work meetings. English may be seen to be more dominant for hard-of-hearing children because we have more opportunity to develop speech, but in reality we could have two equal languages. After all, the government is driving through its social inclusion agenda, and some hearing children are learning BSL if their schools have a sign bilingual or Total Communication policy. Yet hard-of-hearing children, including those with TCS, are cruelly discriminated against. This policy of monolingualism for most deaf children runs counter to the Human Rights Act 1999, the Children Act 1989, the UN Convention on the Rights of the Child (1989) and the Salamanca Statement (1995). These laws and regulations all state that children have a right for their needs to be respected, to a culture, freedom of association and freedom of expression. Hard-of-hearing children, therefore, are in limbo between the two worlds of the Deaf community and hearing society. Jones (1995, 1996) discussed the need for a positive Deaf identity and how hard it is to be Deaf if one has been exposed to the normalization process, so that we are forced to have a think-hearing identity.

In addition, if they do manage to find their way 'home' to the Deaf community, they have to make the transition to being Deaf in later life, by working through the pain of change (Emery, 1999). Emery states that deaf people who have been normalized in Deaf oral schools or mainstream education have to work through the four main stages of acceptance of their Deaf identity: the statis stage, self-conflict, breakthrough and, finally, acceptance.

As with any other community, information is needed by members in order to accept new people into the community. The Deaf community is aware there are some Deaf members who look different or have additional needs, i.e. people with Waardenberg, Klippel–Feil or Usher syndromes, as all of these are usually linked to profound deafness. TCS is relatively unknown in the Deaf community, as few who have it are severely or profoundly Deaf. However, I have been informed that I have a mixed loss of sensorineural and conductive deafness, and that I have become progressively deaf. Nevertheless, I do not feel deafer than I was in childhood; this could be due to audiological advances, or to improved coping abilities. There are still many unanswered questions about TCS, and with respect to deafness itself, particularly the long-term effects of use of technological aids.

Genetic research

Having a disability that is multifaceted and has varying degrees of 'severity' has made me ambivalent about genetic research into the syndrome. My condition, I understand, is still not as limiting as for some people who have TCS. I am said to have mild craniofacial symptoms of the condition, in that my face and jaw are hardly affected, so that I have not needed medical intervention to assist my breathing. The onset of asthma in my late twenties highlighted the problems I had due to the TCS, so that I have required hospitalization and high levels of medical support. As I have grown older, having TCS and asthma has meant that I have had to slow down more quickly than able-bodied peers to a more sedentary life, or else risk hospitalization or long periods of illness. All my life I recall having endless 'colds' and sinusitis which now appear to be linked to rhinitis and allergies, so that, although I enjoyed sports and an active life in my youth, I did unfortunately have after-effects, with extreme tiredness and flu-like symptoms, which spoiled my pleasure somewhat.

> Parents have to accept that there are no guaranteed products on the market that will cure their child's disability. Fortunately, medical attention is devoted to research, giving hope to doctors, families and individuals with disabilities (Davis, 2003).

My main reason for being ambivalent about genetic research is that TCS can be a life-threatening illness or disability, in addition to causing deafness. The breathing problems that accompany TCS can determine a child's ability to breathe unaccompanied, and this obviously affects quality of life. In this case, I think that genetic research is needed to give us more information about the type of gene, how frequently it is found, the odds of it occurring, how much it will affect the quality of life of individuals having it and about treatment. Adults with TCS need to be able to share, and compare the long-term effects of our condition, and this would enable the existing family support group to inform families and maybe offer hope.

My niece is a genetic researcher into cancer, and she expressed an interest in researching deafness instead, as she herself appears to have some of the facial features of TCS. After some deliberation, she and I agreed that 'splitting the DNA' is ethical where it intervenes in life-threatening diseases or disabilities, but not for deafness alone. On the other hand, she felt that, if she had been forewarned during pregnancy that her baby would be deaf, she would then have learned to sign straight away.

All the major features of TCS can be detected by week 15 of embryonic development (Goodrich and Hall, 1995, cited in Davis, 2003) so those mothers who suspect they may be carriers can have prenatal tests. For those who are unaware of their family's genetic make-up, chronic villus sampling or amniocentesis can be offered in weeks 10–18 of pregnancy.

Davis (2003) points out that although 'researchers are developing tests that will aid in more accurate prenatal and postnatal diagnosis of affected individuals, . . . the medical professionals cannot use the genetic tests to predict the severity of an individual's condition'. However, such tests can prepare parents to understand their child's needs as soon as possible.

Predictions about syndromes when a child is in the womb should never be a reason for a termination of a pregnancy, unless there is a grave risk to the mother or the baby, which as yet cannot be proved with TCS. Society has to learn that disability is a celebration of a difference, particularly when it brings with it the richness of culture and languages, as it does with deafness.

Conclusion

We have to cast aside all the negative terms that are linked to genetic syndromes, as they lead to negative self concepts about oneself. I like the term 'dominant gene', as this suggests strength. I certainly do not feel comfortable with the word 'mutant' even though the 'mutant turtles' of the 1990s seemed to take some of the sting out of it! Because of the low prevalence of rare syndromes, we are usually treated like a freak show by the medical profession, and not given the respect we deserve. We are not the 'sufferers' we are often labelled, but humans with dignity.

Knowing that your soul is housed in a body that is different from the norm, and that this makes you whom you are, is the key to acceptance, whether it is deafness alone, or a combined disability. If we are truly proud to be Deaf we must also take in all the other aspects of our deafness; this is an important part of being Deaf.

References

Ballantyne J (1970) Deafness, 2nd edn. Churchill, London, p. 46.

Goodrich JT, Hall CD (1995) Craniofacial anomalies. In: Murphy P (ed.) Growth and Development from a Surgical Perspective. Thième Verlag, New York.

Corker M (1996) Deaf Transitions. Jessica Kingsley Publishers, London.

Davis E (2003) http://freespace.virgin.net/tcs.london/info/edavis.htm.

Emery S (1999) Working through the pain of change. In: Deaf Ex-Mainstreamers' Group (ed.) Between a Rock and a Hard Place: the deaf mainstream experience. Biddles, King's Lynn, pp. 11–13.

Gibbin KP (1988) Otological considerations in the first five years of life. In: McCormick B (ed) Paediatric Audiology 0 to 5 Years. Whurr, London, pp. 37–68.

Jones J (1995) Making the transition to becoming deaf. Deafness 11(1): 4–8.

Jones J (1996) Bilingualism and deaf identity. In: Laurenzi C, Ridgeway S (eds) Progress through Equality. British Society for Mental Health and Deafness, London, pp. 15–20.

NORD (1999) Rare Disease Database [Electronic Database]. National Organization for Rare Disorders, New Fairfield, CT.

Glossary

These definitions are based largely on the words used by deaf people themselves rather than using the medical definitions based on severity and age of onset. In addition, some terms from Read (2001), WHO (2001) and Stephens (1996) have been included.

Activity limitations Difficulties an individual may have in executing activities. Formerly referred to as 'disabilities'.

Audiological physician A medical practitioner specially trained in the diagnosis and non-surgical treatment of patients with hearing and balance disorders.

Audiological scientist A non-medical individual with a master's degree in audiology, concerned with the testing and instrumental management of people with hearing and balance disorders.

Audiological technician (audiologist) A non-medical individual with technical training or a bachelor's degree, concerned with the testing and instrumental aiding of people with hearing and balance disorders.

Audiologist A term applied to different types of professionals with different training in different countries. It leads to confusion and should be avoided.

Auditory brain-stem implant An electromagnetic device inserted into the brain stem of individuals with no cochlear nerves but with a functional auditory system above this level. The principle is that it stimulates the area of the dorsal cochlear nucleus in the brain stem.

Cochlear implant An electromagnetic device inserted surgically into the inner ear of people with limited or no cochlear function, but an intact cochlear nerve. It is intended to stimulate the cochlear nerve.

Deaf (upper case) Denotes those people who see themselves as a part of the Deaf Community, use a National Sign Language and see themselves as part of a linguistic minority.

deaf (lower case) A generic term for all deaf people or for those for whom deafness is perceived as largely audiological without the sociological implications.

Deafblind (as one word) People with severe visual and hearing impairment, who describe themselves as relating to the Deaf world. See also **Dual sensory impairment.**

Deafened People who become profoundly deaf:

- those who become deaf (as opposed to those who are deaf from early childhood)
- other definitions include Sign Language users and those who use speech, lip-reading and/or amplification (sometimes called oral in the literature).

Dual sensory impairment A term used in addition to deafblind for those with some useful sight or hearing.

Environmental factors The physical, social and attitudinal environment in which people live and conduct their lives and which have an effect on deaf people's lives, e.g. the lack of visual information at railway stations or in doctor's surgeries.

Familial Tending to run in families (for genetic or other reasons).

Gene A unit of inheritance containing 'instructions' as to how the body will develop.

Genetic counsellor A health professional giving information and support to individuals and families about conditions or illness that might be genetic in origin.

Hard of hearing Those with some useful hearing who use speech and rely on amplification.

Hearing impaired Can also be used interchangeably with hard of hearing, as a generic term, although its use by professionals covers the full range of hearing levels. This word was previously much disliked by Deaf people but has come back into use through the political disability movement which distinguishes between disability as the social effects of impairment (e.g. lack of access) and the impairment (e.g. the not being able to hear). See also **Social model of disability**.

Hearing impairment Defective function of the auditory system which may be measured using psychoacoustical or physiological techniques.

Hearing therapist A health professional trained to work with people about living with a hearing loss; this may include hearing tactics, working with families and employers.

Hereditary Transmitted by genetic means.

Lip-reading teacher An individual trained to help people to learn to lip-read speech and maximize the hearing they have by focusing on lip patterns and the context of sentences.

Mainstreaming/integration/inclusion Deaf children being educated together with hearing children, as opposed to **segregation** when deaf

children are educated separately, for example in residential schools for
deaf children.

National Sign Language teacher A teacher trained to teach the national
sign language to both deaf and hearing people. They are usually deaf
themselves, native Sign Language users with qualifications in both
language and teaching.

Oralism Education based on speech, lip-reading, amplification and text.

Otolaryngologist A surgeon trained in the diagnosis and treatment of
patients with ear, nose and throat disorders.

Personal factors The particular background of an individual's life and
living, composed of features of the individual that are not part of a
health condition or health state.

Participation restrictions Problems an individual may experience in
involvement in life situations (formerly referred to as 'handicaps').

Social model of disability This implies the recognition of the disadvantages and discrimination experienced as a result of having an impairment (e.g. not being able to attend an education course because of a
lack of accessible provision). This is as opposed to the **medical model
of impairment** which tends to focus on the impairment itself rather
than changing society in order to accommodate the effects of the
impairment and removing the barriers to participation.

Speech and language therapist A person trained to work with the development and rehabilitation of speech and communication. They may
work with deaf children and their families on audiological training or
with people who have had a stroke and suffer from aphasia, for
example.

References

Read A (2001) Genetic terms. In: Martini A, Mazzoli M, Stephens D, Read A (eds)
Definitions, Protocols and Guidelines in Genetic Hearing Impairment. Whurr,
London, pp. 20–25.

Stephens D (1996) Audiological terms. European Workgroup on Genetics of Hearing
Impairment Infoletter 2: 8–9.

WHO (2001) International Classification of Functioning, Disability and Health – ICF.
World Health Organization, Geneva, Switzerland.

Index